*Gender Studies*

# FERTILITY BEHAVIOUR

## POPULATION AND SOCIETY IN A RAJASTHAN VILLAGE

Second Edition

*by*

TULSI PATEL

OXFORD
UNIVERSITY PRESS

OXFORD
UNIVERSITY PRESS

YMCA Library Building, Jai Singh Road, New Delhi 110 001

Oxford University Press is a department of the University of Oxford. It furthers the University's objective of excellence in research, scholarship, and education by publishing worldwide in

Oxford New York
Auckland Cape Town Dar es Salaam Hong Kong Karachi
Kuala Lumpur Madrid Melbourne Mexico City Nairobi
New Delhi Shanghai Taipei Toronto

With offices in
Argentina Austria Brazil Chile Czech Republic France Greece
Guatemala Hungary Italy Japan Poland Portugal Singapore
South Korea Switzerland Thailand Turkey Ukraine Vietnam

Oxford is a registered trade mark of Oxford University Press in the UK and in certain other countries

Published in India by Oxford University Press, New Delhi



First published 1994
Second edition 2006



ISBN 13: 978-0-19-568706-4
ISBN 10: 0-19-568706-X

Typeset in AGaramond 10.5/12 at S.R.Enterprises
Printed in India at De-Unique, New Delhi-110018
Published by Oxford University Press
YMCA Library Building, Jai Singh Road, New Delhi 110 001

FERTILITY BEHAVIOUR

To
Bāi and Papa

# Contents

MAPS

# Acknowledgements

I am extremely grateful to Professor A. M. Shah for his unstinted guidance throughout this research. Thanks also to Professor B. N. Nanda, M. Anjum, M. Z. Khan Dr B. S. Nagi, Dr S. Hemraj, A. S. Kohli, Ravi Kapoor, Qamar Agha, Biswajeet Das, K. J. Geetha, Mani Arulnandhi, Nishat Qaiser, Shakeel Ahmed, Kusum Sharma, Sheena Jain, S. Zainuddin, N. H. Zuberi and N. K. Nijhawan. The staff of Zakhir Hussain library and the faculties of natural-and Bio-sciences departments of Jamia Millia Islamia deserve my gratitude. I am thankful to Dr S. Z. Qasim, Vice-Chancellor, Jamia Millia Islamia, for his encouragement. For special thanks I must single out Mohmmad Talib who offered valuable help. I deeply acknowledge the encouragement and advice given by Professors A. Minocha, B. S. Baviskar, E. A. Ramaswamy, Dr Khadija Gupta, Gopal Bhardwaj and in particular Dr Uma Ramaswamy.

I must thank the staff of Ratan Tata Library. The members of its processing section and Rama Aggarwal, in particular, were helpful in various ways. I am indebted to the Indian Council of Socience Research for bearing part of my research expenses.

The people of Mogra will remain dear to me. My special thanks go to Bagta Ramji (*Kaka*). It would be impossible to itemize my indebtedness to my parents, sistors, brothers, *babhi* and other family members who contributed in various ways to the progress of my research. I could not have completed my work without the immense help I received from my husband Radheshyam, son Vinay and daughter Savita.

# A Note on Transliteration

Diacritical marks are used to indicate pronunciation of local words. However, names of persons, groups, places and terms whose use is accepted in Sociology and in Indian English, such as *jati, dai, jajmani, khalsa, bapu, patwari, purdah* and panchayat are spelt without diacritical marks. Long vowels are indicated by a dash over the letters where they occur at the beginning or in the middle of a word. For example, *akro* is pronounced as *aakro*. This diacritical mark is, however, dropped for the last letter of a word, because such vowel endings tend invariably to be elongated. In some cases where the last vowel sound is exceptionally elongated, two letters of the vowel are used to indicate the phonetic difference.

*Vowels*

| *Short* | *Long* | *Pronounced approximately as in* | |
|---|---|---|---|
| a | ā | up | ask |
| i | ī | in | eat |
| u | ū | put | boot |
| e | ē | egg | ale |
| o | ō | gone | go |

I have spelt stressed consonants by doubling the letter, for example, *punna* to stress the letter 'n'. However, I have not attempted to distinguish hard and soft consonants when they are at the beginning of a word. Frequently, such consonants are hard. Retroflexes are indexed by placing a dot beneath the letter, for example ḍ, ḷ, ṇ.

# *Preface to the Second Edition*

I am delighted to write this preface as it provides me the opportunity to express my indebtedness to two sets of readers and owe them thanks. The first set of readers include my students in universities in Delhi and abroad, who have over the years given me feedback on this book. The book was sold out both in Indian and foreign markets within the first few years of its publication. I was on a commonwealth fellowship at the London School of Economics, London in 1996–7 and the copies in the UK sold out within a few weeks of the talks I gave on my research.

Of late, the relationship between anthropology and demography has begun to be respected in India as well after it has been valued in the Western academia for over a decade. The second set of readers are scholars who have pursued their research interest in fertility studies, and those who have consciously tried to blur the boundaries between demography and anthropology. This book was already published in 1994 when Greenhalgh's (1995) call for 'structuration' and 'practice' theories in demography were being made in the US, where she called for 'whole demographies' of villages and communities. Fertility studies in general have also provided me an opportunity to look at them in retrospect, which I provide in the introduction to this edition. I am fortunate to have unstinting professional advice from Professor A.M. Shah and I am grateful to him.

I must acknowledge the warm and forthcoming interaction I had with the editors at Oxford University Press. I cannot thank them enough, for not only sharing warmly the processes of the project but also for patiently bearing with me while I took time to complete the introduction. I would like to thank my husband, R.S. Patel and daughter, Savita Patel, even though it is not enough to just acknowledge their cooperation and support.

New Delhi
21 July 2006

TULSI PATEL

# Preface

Population growth, especially fertility trends, continue to pose major dilemmas for policy makers, administrators, researchers and others the world over, more particularly in the third world. Since the early 60s there has been a marked increase both in the quantity and quality of research dealing with India's population, and particularly fertility determinants, differentials and change.

Over 70% of the Indian population resides in villages, which constitute the basic units of structure. Rajasthan figures amongst the preponderantly rural states. Also, population wise, it is one of the five problem states, others being Uttar Pradesh, Madhya Pradesh, Bihar and Orissa. Therefore, a holistic study of fertility behaviour in a village named Mogra in western Rajasthan was undertaken. The study was earlier submitted as a dissertation for the award of Ph.D. at the university of Delhi, India.

The present study attempts to advance the sociological knowledge of fertility behaviour based on field study in a village. It is realised only recently that intensive community studies are needed to understand comprehensively an intimate behaviour like human fertility. There is a paucity of studies, both in India and outside it, providing an in-depth understanding of human fertility behaviour. This study tries to fill this gap by observing fertility behaviour not only in the context of other demographic factors such as sex, age and mortality but also the social system in general. Based on the participant observation method, a census of the village, retrospective fertility histories of all ever married women in the village, genealogies, and case studies of men and women, the study presents dense description and interpretive account of fertility behaviour. This is thus a contribution in the field of micro-level, holistic, indepth studies of fertility behaviour. It belongs to the only now emerging genre of research that combines anthropology, demography and sociology.

This thesis reviews some of the controversies in demographic literature in the light of data from the field study village. It attempts to highlight the view that, instead of measuring directly the impact of socioeconomic factors on fertility, substantial insights are gained in exploring and analysing the specific institutional mechanisms through which socioeconomic factors operate.

The study explores how the objective conditions of life, including the emergent change, are linked with people's subjective orientations, including values and norms of fertility behaviour. Giddens' (1984) concept of 'duality of structure' has been the theoretical tool for understanding fertility behaviour in this study. It analyses the institutional mechanisms and customary activities and norms helping to regulate and socially reproduce over time the fertilitybehaviour. Giddens' (1984) concept of 'structuration' is deployed in the understanding of the management, regulation, and social reproduction of fertility behaviour. In other words, the couples employ the rules and resources to recreate the very structures through which they represent themselves as actors.

Finally, the concept of 'fertility career' of a couple is critical to understand the social regulation of fertility behaviour as a process rather than as a static phenomenon. The developmental process of the household (Shah 1973) has heuristic value in the understanding of the developmental phases of the fertility career of a couple.

Tulsi Patel
Delhi, 1994

# *Introduction to the Second Edition*

Fertility forms an important cornerstone of national as well as international concerns regarding numerous aspects of human life as well as the environment. During the latter part of the 20th century, one of the three main processes of population, fertility which has more than the other two processes, that is, mortality and migration, attracted attention for research and policy purposes.

In the modern era, population has a history of debate among academic circles and public policy-makers. Malthus's debate with Godwin and Condorcet regarding the well-being of human populations goes back to the 18th century. The poor Laws debate, the Neo-Malthusian League, and the latter's regional wings in the late 19th and early 20th centuries are examples of the importance given to the size of population and its relationship with inequality and well-being in most countries in the world.

In the last six decades, especially since World War II, fertility gained central importance when international aid and assistance agencies started to intervene and influence the population policies of newly emerged Third World countries. Warnings were issued in subtle and not so subtle ways by international population institutes and development aid agencies to control the rate of fertility and population growth beginning with the end of World War II. Having got acceptance as a social science in the American academia, demography began to establish itself as a discipline only in the 1920s and 1930s, and did not take long to grapple with the problem of high fertility, especially in the context of the Cold War scenario.

However, historically speaking, mortality, more than fertility, has been of greater concern in matters of population. Guha's (2001) recapitulation of population changes since the Neolithic revolution highlights that while fertility may be the central problem for contemporary demography, historical studies must give equal or greater weightage to mortality. Harris (1968) had referred to the prominent French savant Holbach who proposed a cyclical moral economy of reproduction, in which luxury lapses into tyranny, followed by depopulation and consequent fall of empires, and a return to virtues of high fertility and repopulation. For South Asian population, Guha (2001) observes that high mortality led to stable populations or a slower rate of population growth in many parts of the world until it grew rapidly in the modern era of the Industrial Revolution. Based on an extensive review of historical demographic studies he argues that an explanation of population growth must be an explanation of mortality decline in the early 20th century. Different views have been provided for the reasons of mortality decline. While one view holds decline in morbidity and mortality to improvement in nutritional status of the population prior to the availability of effective therapies against infections until World War II, the other holds, among others, the rise of people's immunities because of changes in host–parasite relations. Mortality was paid attention in the essays by Habib (1982) and Visaria and Visaria (1982) on the patterns of population growth in India, and Davis (1951) in his account of the population of India and Pakistan.

It is little wonder that Dyson (1989) in his edited volume on India's historical demography regretted the paucity of research and remarked that the historical demography of India as a field of inquiry hardly exists. In the present context, historical demography provides an important input to understand the swift turn of focus from mortality and slow growing populations to the fast growing ones in recent decades; and subsequently more attention to fertility.

It is a daunting task to cover the whole spectrum of research on fertility, after World War II, given the quantum of empirical research published. I shall recapitulate some of the salient trends, patterns, and shifts in interest discernible in the studies on fertility in India over the last few decades. Having outlined the important demographic conceptual and theoretical contributions with respect to population growth in the introduction of this edition first published in 1994, I shall elaborate on the classical theory of demographic transition, the fountainspring of most of fertility and family planning studies. The earlier introduction has been retained for the reader interested in how ethnography of a village is located in the context of the existing fertility studies.

## I

For most of the latter part of twentieth century, population growth was seen from the modernization and development paradigm as it were. Modernism as a Western movement is expressed as a number of tendencies in thought and practice. Modernity and modernization in social anthropology was also, like in many other social sciences, derived from the second half of the 19th century, making a distinction between the present age (modern) and the past. The theory of Demographic Transition (Thompson 1929; Notestein 1945) inspired by this view, was applied to population and fertility studies. The theory is based on the idea of social and economic inequalities and a unilinear path of development. Countries with lower industrial growth are less socially developed and thus have higher fertility even after their mortality has been curtailed. The emerging bulge in population of those countries owing to sustained high fertility is a cause for concern (for more on this, see Patel and Purewal 2005).

Population thus enters into and complicates the neat 'growth versus equity' trade off equation. For a country to continue to mark economic growth and development, its population needs to balance in a manner so that savings after consumption may be set aside to be ploughed back as investment, besides resources for increasing capacity of people to enhance labour productivity. This population–resources balance is conveyed in economics and demography through the concept of optimum population. Paul Ehrlich's book, *The Population Bomb* (1968) sent danger signals that overpopulation would result in inadequate resources to sustain the human population. The correlation between overpopulation and resources points to population increases globally, particularly the uneven rates of population growth in the context of the earth's resources, which are argued to be finite.

A spate of studies, influenced by the theory of demographic transition, explored the causes and proximate determinants of fertility as well as family planning in the 1960s and 1970s, the golden period in demography. Many of the studies were funded by international population institutions, such as Population Council, International Planned Parenthood Federation, Ford Foundation, and also the World Bank (see Ross 1998). Local governments too supported many other studies on fertility and family planning. A number of journals on population, such as *Demography*, the flag ship in the discipline, and *Population and Development Review* in the United States, *Population Studies* in England, *Population* and *Genus* in France, and many more in other parts of Europe were set up to publish demographic studies. *Demography India* is fairly a recent journal. Demographic trends and projections and statistical sophistication received an impetus in these publications. Besides the many national associations for population studies, international professional bodies like the International Union of Population Studies (IUSSP) established since 1928 enabled a number of scholars to publish their studies as authored and edited volumes. Large-scale surveys like the World Fertility Survey of the 1970s and Demographic and Health Surveys of the 1980s and 1990s were conducted across several countries. India participated in these surveys at a later stage, and the two phases of National Family and Health Surveys (NFHS I of 1992–93 and II of 1998–99) provide data for demographic studies.

But today, the demographic transition's unilear view of population equation through the play of fertility and mortality is no longer a unanimously accepted route. Even a simple economic calculus for development does not hold good for many economies. Osmani (2001) has detailed the empirical inadequacy of the view linking capital accumulation with growth. Some of the world's most populated countries with high fertility have experienced high rates of growth in per capita income in recent decades. These countries are India, Indonesia, Pakistan, Thailand, Turkey, Korea, China, with the exception of some sub-Saharan African ones. Cassen (1994) clearly points out the inconclusive, if not entirely negative, evidence of several studies questioning the inverse relationship between population growth and economic development.

Further, rapid fertility transitions have been observed in a majority of developing countries for over three decades. Between the early 1960s to the late 1980s, the total fertility rate of the developing world declined by an estimated 36 per cent—from 6.0 to 3.8 births per woman (UN 1995). Demographers have been grappling with this transformation in terms of looking for an argument that holds good theoretically as well as empirically. This, however, is not a new phenomenon. Since the Ansley Coale led Princeton European Fertility Project, which began in 1963, demographic thesis of synchrony between socio-economic development and fertility decline has been shaken. The classic predictors of fertility decline offered by the theory of demographic transition failed to account for the historic decline in fertility. Declining fertility trends in economically disparate nations on the one hand and the booming economies of highly populated China and India have posed a serious challenge to theory in demography. In addition, the latter two countries' experiences have brought about a major shift in the attitude that fertility is a problem in itself, that is, a hurdle in development. This shift in view is seen in the admiration for the potential of large working age populations in India and China. The IUSSP has, a couple of years ago, proposed to revise one of its aims by deleting the word 'problem' and stressing on the analyses of population 'processes'.

## II

When *Fertiltiy Behaviour* was published in 1994, village demographies in India were non-existent. A very large number of KAP (knowledge, attitude, and practice) surveys on fertility and family planning were sponsored and published on Indian society. They applied social science and demographic knowledge to curtail the teeming millions who were responsible for the underdevelopment of the country, a clear influence of the demographic transition theory. Nehru (1958) in one of his speeches mentioned that he had 380 million problems as India had 380 million people. The studies were to supply information to enable policy intervention for fertility control. Rao (1974) had reviewed 550 such KAP studies on fertility, family planning, and contraceptive practice during 1951–74. She found that most studies had used interview-schedules or questionnaires with the exception of two that had used observation as a method. Though Rao was less than appreciative of the theoretical and conceptual inputs of such studies, their import in the 1970s and 1980s had continued.

Sociological studies on fertility in India, scant though these were, began to appear by mid-1970s. D.G. Mandelbaum, an anthropologist from California, Berkeley published his study in 1974, *Human Fertility in India*, exploring the factors affecting population growth in India. His study was based on a variety of source materials. A few papers in the edited volumes by Jongman and Cleassen (1974) and Tien and Bien (1974) explored factors that other surveys had not considered. Three years later, Srinivas and Ramaswamy (1977) in *Culture and Human Fertility in India*, based on secondary data from Indian village studies picked out interesting sociological pointers to fertility behaviour. These village studies were published until the mid-1970s. Village studies in India had begun with S.C. Dube's *Indian Village* (1955), McKim Marriott *Village India* (1955) and M.N. Srininvas's *India's Villages* (1955). The peak in village studies continued in the 1960s and 1970s, conducted by anthropologists from the US, the UK, and India. Many were particularly encouraged by Srinivas who had set up the department of sociology at the Delhi School of Economics in 1958–9 after his Oxford and Baroda days. A few studies not fitting exactly into the category of village studies, but which had fertility and family planning as their central focus, were also drawn upon as data source. It is a strange coincidence that though village studies in India had their golden period roughly during the same period as demographic studies on fertility transition—from mid-1950s to mid-1970s—there was little communication between the two genres.

Village studies were carried out with a different intent, given the fieldwork tradition and holistic approach of social anthropology, Their stress on describing village society and culture provided the ethnography from which issues pertaining to fertility behaviour could be expected. Srinivas and Ramaswamy's (1977) small book culled out some of the salient linkages with fertility in village India that had not been raised by earlier fertility studies. Papers in Epstein and Jackson's (1977) edited volume on the feasibility of fertility planning came out at the same time. Five years later, subsequent to Dyson and Moore's (1983) paper on kinship and fertility differentials between north and south India, demographic studies incorporated culture as a variable into fertility. Basu's 1992 study is among the earliest serious attempts. Though anthropologists like Nag (1972 and 1978) and Das Gupta (1987) had earlier taken up the issue of incorporating society and culture into fertility, fertility studies were mostly questionnaire-oriented and ahistorical. Nor were there any village-based holistic studies on fertility in India, as we shall see in the last section. The focus on women between the ages 15 and 45 only speaks about the concern with the present.

## III

Woman as a child bearer is an important constituent in fertility studies. Most fertility measures are based with women in the reproductive age as the denominator. Demographic studies in India have paid attention to women merely as bearers and rearers of children, and as potential users of contraception to curtail fertility. Derived from the theory of demographic transition, the assumption was if women were modern they would use contraception and plan their families. The eurocentric perspective of modernity in women expected them to possess modern indicators, such as education, employment, income, etc., on which depended their fertility reduction efforts. Gathering information with laudable objectives of development and well-being, fertility studies were conducted with the intent to inform policy. Besides, most contraceptives were oriented towards the female; and feminist women were also the ones to demand birth control at the turn of 20th century (for feminists on birth control and population control, see Patel and Purewal 2005).

At an aggregate level, demographic studies found modern women more knowledgeable about contraception and assumed they had higher status than those with higher fertility (Mason 1984). Status of women based on modernity indicators was treated as a variable in itself, as though it is derived in isolation from their social and cultural context.

For a discussion of the socially and culturally situated status of women see Chapters 3 and 7 in this book. 'Different definitions of the status of women imply a comparison with the status of men. Women's rights (Dixon 1975), women's status (Dixon 1978), patriarchy (Cain *et al.* 1979), men's situational advantage (Caldwell 1981), female power and autonomy (Safilios-Rothschild 1982), female autonomy (Dyson and Moore 1983)' (Patel 2004: 208; see this paper for an extended discussion on status of women and for 'women's autonomy' in demographic studies. Also see Madhok's (2004) scholarly discussion on women in demography). In 1993 Mason used the term 'position' of women. Many other papers in the same edited collection used the concepts of 'status' and 'position' against empirical data from different societies. The term 'status' was dropped in favour of the term women's 'autonomy' deployed in demographic studies by Dyson and Moore (1983). Later, several studies, including Jejeebhoy (1995) and the collection of essays on education of women and fertility edited by Jeffery and Basu (1996) preferred the term 'autonomy' to 'status'. Empirical research has shown diverse trends in the education of women and their fertility rather than a convincing theory of fertility decline. Murthi and Dreze (1999) raised some complex issues emerging out of education and development in relation to fertility.

My study (1994) found that fertility, especially a son's birth, improved a woman's status, and only after having grown up children, including of course sons, a woman attains higher status and is then enabled to negotiate with the concerned others, her wish to arrest her fertility (see also Patel [1999] and the notion of a social optimum number of children). In short, while fertility influences a young bride's status at one point, it is her status as a mother of grown ups that influences her fertility later on.

When demographic studies attempt correlations between the number of children born to a woman or couple and variables of modernization and development, such as education, income, occupation, family type, the finer meaning of childbirth to a mother/father/other kin gets lost in statistical aggregations. The semiotic depth of each child's birth by parity and sex of the baby for the mother, who not only begets the baby, but is also situated in the midst of her household and familial ties, is not static. There are socially prevalent notions about when to begin, when to end, and how many children of what sex are ideal to have. Therefore, the relevance of data on how each of the births is organized and how the kins respond to these events. The response of the significant others means a lot to the mother, as does her fertility performance to the family and the community. This field of meaning and symbols is more a topic for anthropological rather than demographic studies. McCormack (1982), Patel (1982), Blanchet (1984), Jeffery *et al.* (1989), Chawla (1994) discuss the social and cultural organization of childbirth, participation of many during birth, post-partum and afterwards. This book sees the interlinkages between births and social relations through which women's status is built and socially constructed. In status considerations it is always what is socially desirable and valuable that gets accounted, and this holds for fertility as well. Closer observation of societal processes is a methodological provision to notice the play of subtler social processes. As early as 1927, Mayo had found how the birth of a son brings an air of authority and confidence in a meek young bride in Bengal.

Gender considerations within the life cycle of the woman at different stations in her life, and in her relationship in the household and the family come to weave a tapestry of a certain fertility pattern which was rarely found in demographic studies (Patel 1982). Watkins had earlier (1993) raised the question of how much we know about women from the large number of demographic studies. This issue remains unresolved in fertility studies and more so because not only does a woman's status vary cross-culturally, it is fluid within cultures and for an individual during her life cycle. In this book, I adopted the life cycle perspective to explore fertility behaviour of women over time. While the priorities, wants, and desires shift and are modified in the process of family building experiences of individual couples and those around them, child mortality within and outside the household is perceived to be an important ingredient in fertility decisions over the life cycle. This fluidity of a moving preference for the number of children based on a series of a person's and others' fertility as well as child mortality (not just infant mortality which is correlated with fertility in demographic studies) experiences is yet to be incorporated into demographic theory. The chapter on child mortality in this book discusses the meaning of infant and child mortality to mothers, the household, and the family, and is not limited to the meaning it has for persons in the reproductive age alone. It brings out the interactions in which fertility and child mortality experiences of parents, aunts, mothers-in-law, and even neighbours and friends are taken into account which in turn influence fertility considerations. The semiotics of the larger ambience surrounding a reproductive couple is methodologically and theoretically significant for studies on fertility and changes therein.

Women belong to families and households and their reproductive behaviour is organized in a cultural and social context. Srinivas and Ramaswamy (1977) highlighted this aspect of women's lives in Indian village studies, thus moving beyond correlations of fertility with age at marriage, its duration, residence, marriage patterns, etc. Gender was incorporated into their studies by the historian Clark (1989, 1993) for the Patidar and Koli communities in Gujarat, and Das Gupta (1987), the demographer-cum-anthropologist, on selective discrimination of daughters in Punjab. These have been ground-breaking studies, especially in the light of the alarmingly skewed sex ratio figures in India at present, more glaringly visible in the 0–6 year age group. The decreasing proportion of girls is now apparent in the sex composition in elementary schools in India, and the difficulty many boys face in finding brides in regions worst affected by sex selective abortions. This trend in South and Southeast Asia seriously questions the relationship of gender with advances in reproductive science and socio-economic development. For an extensive coverage on different aspects of female foeticide, see Patel (forthcoming).

Reproductive rights and reproductive choice (Hartman 1987) have gained greater prominence in the 1990s build up towards the International Conference on Population and Development in Cairo. Feminists debates with the pro-life and pro-choice positions on reproduction, and the earlier focus on the body and medicalization of birth have been attracting more research, political, and policy attention, thus posing a crisis for the conventional demographic methods and conceptual frameworks. The collection of essays in Ginsburg and Rapp

(1995) and Davis-Floyd and Sargent (1997) are a few among the large number of studies on the anthropology of the politics of reproduction (for more on this issue see Introduction it, Patel, forthcoming).

## IV

Demographic research is designed to collect quantifiable data that yield to correlations. Individuals are aggregated to explain their behaviour. But individual decision-making might itself be produced by the form and content of relationships among individuals mediated by the nature of symbols through which they communicate. It is here that most KAP and correlation studies of fertility can be seen to exhibit the limitations of methodological individualism.

Methodologically demography's concern has been for mathematical precision based on large data sets. Many fertility studies mentioned earlier had correlated fertility with socio-economic, and more recently, the preference for sons. Explanations can be found for any correlation. For intimate matters like fertility behaviour, studies following demographic methodology encounter serious limitations, which were realized especially in the 1990s with unanticipated fertility transitions occurring in several disparate societies. While community and small-scale fieldwork-based social anthropological studies provide concepts, demography's preference is to deploy the concepts to large areas and numbers. Though there is sharing, there is also discord between the methods of the two disciplines and demography laments that their field is all methods and no theory (Greenhalgh 1995). Individuals are important and cannot be lost sight of. It was much later in the day when I discovered that one household with a couple, their five sons, and a widowed mother (of the head of household) were inadvertently left out of the numerical calculation in the household census of the village in the first edition of this book. While this is entirely my shortcoming, it need not be viewed as a limitation of the anthropological method.

The dichotomy between the terms 'behaviour' and 'action' as unintentional and intentional acts respectively, is a problem in social science. By using the term behaviour, one is using a wider pantheon of human activity, including specific behaviour, habit (sociogenic), and action (intentional). New directions research could be found by working out the methodological procedures and theoretical relationship between individual behaviour and larger social processes. Don't we all know very well that most of us act and behave keeping our position and status in mind? The reflexive and knowledgeable people studied in fertility research are no different, as in this book.

## V

During the last two decades, anthropology and demography have begun to speak with each other at the self-reflective initiative by demographers themselves. Caldwell *et al.* (1987 and 1988) insisted on incorporating more anthropology into demographic research. Caldwell, the first to appeal to embrace anthropology, preferred the adoption of anthropological method into demography but with little input from anthropological theory, though his (1982) work on intergenerational wealth flows and fertility was significant. Thus the stress within this genre of demographic research seeks theoretical support to understand why people have the number of children they have. There have been two developments enabling a dialogue across these disciplines. Demographic research has been in search of a theory which can explain the kind of changes taking place in the world in the wake of the onset of fertility transition in most countries as discussed earlier. Cultural institutions in different settings influenced the phenomenon of fertility independently of socio-economic conditions. But culture was eventually treated in fertility studies as a mere variable rather than a complex of meanings of actions and intentions in a given society. Greenhalgh (1995) has discussed the problems of cultural reductionism and of communication in the diffusion approach in demography. While demographic research also continues to be influenced by micro economic considerations and focuses on the individual and/or the couple, sociological connections with social institutions, such as family, kinship, and with macro structures, such as the state, the market, and socio-economic development remain to be teased out.

Second, demography has been opening up to methodological intrusions by other disciplines into its own realm. Demography has been rather accommodative and thus anthropological demography has been institutionalized as a branch of demography rather than of anthropology. Also, the recently more troubling demographic behaviour, both with new reproductive technologies and declining fertility in poorer countries has further motivated demographers to engage in a dialogue with social anthropology, an interaction thought of little worth in earlier times.

The real challenge, however, is to construct whole demographies that illuminate the multi-level and mutually constitutive relations between culture and political economy, and the implications of these relations for reproductive actors (Greenhalgh 1995). Kertzer and Fricke (1997) have provided an informed account of the twin purposes behind the interface between demography and anthropology and a quest for a more sophisticated social and cultural theory. They warn that it is not an exercise meant to 'add fieldwork and stir', with primacy on methodological individualism and quantitative orientation focused on individual level variation. The intent is for an exercise with an interest in meaning and motivation.

There is evidence of slightly more than a couple of attempts of anthropological research on fertility in India. Anthropologists and sociologists have produced ethnographic work either on fertility behaviour and family planning (Mamdani [1972] conducted fieldwork in a village in Punjab though rather hurriedly; Jeffery *et al.* [1989] in two villages in Uttar Pradesh; Patel [1994] used Giddens' structuration thesis in a village in Rajasthan; Jeffery and Jeffery [1997] again used the political economy perspective in the same villages of Uttar Pradesh). Saavala (2001) has used Bourdieu's practice approach to fertility decline in a village in south India. Jeffery and Jeffery (1996) have mentioned these in their work on the everyday life of rural women. While viewing the theoretical and methodological limitations of demographic studies, one must not forget to confront the influence of assumptions on ethnographic description in anthropological studies, whatever the theoretical underpinnings.

The politics of population is not just related to development as in the demographic transition theory. Population has been decisive in the history of many nations and nationalities. The controversies and politics of numbers hold no less significance even today. The demographic size of political constituencies comes up now and again during Indian elections. The political heat generated with the release of demographic data on religion by the 2001 Census was so intense as to roll a few heads. In contrast, no heads rolled after the 2001 Census data on missing girls was released, though a great deal of concern was expressed. This in itself is a matter of grave concern regarding the politics of gender, vote bank, and numbers. Politicization of population is taking place in varying ways in different parts of the world. This is an area of study begging research. At present, issues of public health, reproductive health, and old age are attracting the attention of demographers where partnership with anthropology might be worthwhile. A word of caution, however, may be given. Anthropological fieldwork of the conventional kind where a minimum of one year is spent in the field if not more, besides additional visits, is becoming less fashionable in some anthropological quarters. Going to the field and recording with utmost patience and care every detail about social life through observation, conversation, and other means is not being followed. The touch and go kind of anthropology is gaining popularity. The depth derived from conventional fieldwork-based ethnography has its own value though it comes with a great cost in terms of time, skill, and resources. The future course of sharing between the two disciplines is certain to happen with demography having opened its barriers.

## *References*

Basu, A.M. 1992. *Culture, the Status of Women, and Demographic Behaviour: Illustrated with the Case of India*, Oxford: Clarendon Press.

Blanchet, T. 1984. *Meanings and Rituals of Birth in Rural Bangladesh*, Dhaka: The University Press Ltd.

Cain, M., S.R. Khanam, and S. Nahar. 1979. 'Class, Patriarchy and Women's Work in Bangladesh', *Population and Development Review* 5(3): 405.

Caldwell, J.C. 1981. 'The Mechanisms of Demographic Change in Historical Perspective', *Population Studies*, 35 (1): 5–27.

Caldwell, J.C., P. Caldwell, and B. Caldwell. 1987. 'Anthropology and Demography: The Mutual Reinforcement of Speculation and Research', *Current Anthropology* 28 (1): 25–43.

Caldwell, J.C., P.H. Reddy, and P. Caldwell. 1988. *The Causes of Demographic Change*, Wisconsin: University of Wisconsin Press.

Cassen, R. 1994. *Population and Development: Old Debates, New Conclusions*, Washington, DC: Overseas Development Council.

Chawla, J. 1994. *Child-bearing and Culture: Women Centred Revisioning of the Traditional Midwife, the Dai as a Ritual Practitioner*, Delhi: Indian Social Institute.

Clark, A.W. 1989. 'Mortality, Fertility and Women', in T. Dyson (ed.), *India's Historical Demography*, London: Curzon Press, 119–49.

——. 1993. 'Analysing the Reproductions of Human Beings', in A.W. Clark (ed.), *Gender and Political Economy: Explorations of South Asian Systems*. Delhi: Oxford University Press, pp. 115–45.

Das Gupta, M. 1987. 'Selective Discrimation against Female Children in Rural Punjab, India', *Population and Development Review*, 13(i): 77–100.

Davis, K. 1951. *The Population of India and Pakistan*, Princeton: Princeton University Press.

Davis-Floyd, R.E. and C.F. Sargent (eds). 1997. *Childbirth and Authoritative Knowledge*, California: University of California Press.

Dixon, R.B. 1975. *Women's Rights and Fertility: Reports on Population/Family Planning*, New York: The Population Council.

——. 1978. *Rural Women at Work: Strategies for Development in South Asia*, Baltimore: Johns Hopkins University Press.

Dube, S.C. 1955. *Indian Village*, London: Routledge and Kegan Paul.

Dyson, T. (ed.). 1989. *India's Historical Demography*, London: Curzon Press.

Dyson, T. and M. Moore. 1983. 'On Kinship Structure: Female Autonomy and Demographic Behaviour in India', *Population and Development Review*, 9 (10): 35–60.

Ehrlich, P. 1968. *The Population Bomb*, New York: Ballentine Books.

Epstein, S.T. and D. Jackson. 1977. *The Feasibility of Fertility Planning*, London: Pergamon Press.

Ginsburg, F. and R. Rapp (eds). 1995. *Conceiving the New World Order*, Berkeley: University of California Press.

Government of India. 1958. *Jawahar Lal Nehru: Selected Speeches*. 1953-57. Vol. 3, Delhi: Publications Division.

Greenhalgh, S. 1995. *Situating Fertility: Anthropology and Demographic Inquiry*, Cambridge: Cambridge University Press.

Guha, S. 2001. *Health and Population in South Asia*, London: Hurst and Company.

Habib, I. 1982. 'Population', in T. Raychaudhuri and I. Habib (eds), *The Cambridge Economic History of India*, Hyderabad: Orient Longman, Vol 1, 163–71.

Harris, M. 1968. *The Rise of Anthropological Theory*, New York: Routledge and Kegan Paul.

Hartman, B. 1987. *Reproductive Rights and Wrongs: The Global Politics of Population Control and Contraceptive Choice*, New York: Harper and Row.

Jeffery, R. and M.A. Basu (eds). 1996. *Girls' Schooling, Women's Autonomy and Fertility Change in South Asia*, New Delhi: Sage.

Jeffery, P. and R. Jeffery. 1996. *Don't Marry Me to a Ploughman! Women's Everyday Lives in Rural North India*, Boulder: Westview Press.

Jeffery, P. and R. Jeffery. 1997. *Population, Gender and Politics: Demographic Change in Rural India*, Cambridge: Cambridge University Press.

Jejeebhoy, S. 1995. *Women's Education, Autonomy and Reproductive Behaviour: Experience from Developing Countries,* Oxford: Clarendon Press.

Jongman, D.G. and H.J.M. Cleassen (eds). 1974. *The Neglected Factor*, The Netherlands: Van Gorcum and Company.

Kertzer, D. and T. Fricke. 1997. *Anthropological Demography: Toward a New Synthesis*, Chicago: University of Chicago Press.

Madhok, S. 2004. 'Heteronomous women? Hidden Assumptions in the Demography of Women,' in M. Unnithan-Kumar (ed.), *Reproductive Agency, Medicine and the State*, Oxford: Berghahn Books, 223–44.

Mamdani, M. 1972. *The Myth of Population Control*, New York: Monthly Review Press.

Marriott, McKim (ed.). 1955. *Village India*, Chicago: University of Chicago Press.

Mason, K.O. 1984. *The Status of Women: A Review of its Relation to Fertility and Mortality*, New York: The Rockefeller Foundation.

Mason, K.O. 1993. 'The Impact of Women's Position on Demographic Change During the Course of Development,' in N. Federici, K.O. Mason, and S. Sogner (eds), *Women's Position and Demographic Change*, Oxford: Clarendon Press.

Mayo, K. 1927. *Mother India*, Bombay: Allied.

Murthi, M. and J. Dreze. 1999. *Fertility, Education, Development: Further Evidence from India*, Kings College Cambridge: Centre for History and Economics.

Nag, M. 1972. 'Sex Culture and Human Fertility: India and the United States', *Current Anthropology*, 13; 231–7, 260–3.

Nag, M., R.C. Peet, and B.N.F. White. 1978. 'An Anthropological Approach to the Study of the Agronomic Values of Children in Java and Nepal',

*Current Anthropology*, 19: 293–306.

Osmani, S.R. 2001. 'On Equality', in J. Blau (ed.) *Blackwell Companion to Sociology,* Maulden, Mass.: Blackwell Publishers.

Patel, T. 1999. 'The Precious Few: Women's Agency, Household Progression and Fertility in a Rajasthan Village,' *Journal of Comparative Family Studies*, 30 (4): 429–51.

——. 2004. 'Women in Fertility Studies and *In Situ*', in M. Unnithan-Kumar (ed.), *Reproductive Agency, Medicine and the State*, Oxford: Berghahn Books, 203–22.

Patel, T. and T. Purewal. 2005. 'Origins and Contours of the population Debate: Inequality, Population Politics and the Population Debate', in M. Romero and E. Margolis (eds), *The Blackwell Companion to Social Inequalities*, New York: Blackwell, 441–65.

Patel, T. (forthcoming). *Sex Selective Abortion in India: Gender, society and New Reproductive Technologies in India,* New Delhi: Sage.

Rao, K.G. 1974. *Studies in Family Planning: India*, New Delhi: Abhinav.

Ross, E.B. 1998. *The Malthus Factor: Poverty, Politics and Population in Capitalist Development*, London: Zed Books.

Saavala, M. 2001. *Fertility and Familial Power Relations: Procreation in South India*, England: Curzon.

Safilios-Rothschild, C. 1982. 'Female Power, Autonomy and Demographic Change in the Third World', in R. Anker, M. Buvinic, and N.H. Youssef (eds), *Women's Roles and Population Trends in the Third World*, London: Croom Helm.

Srininvas, M.N. (ed.). 1955. *India's Villages,* Bombay: Asia Publishing House.

Tien, H.Y. and F.D. Bien (eds). 1974. *Comparative Family and Fertility Research*, Leiden: E.J. Brill.

United Nations. 1995. *Human Development Report 1995*, New York: UNDP.

Visaria, P. and L. Visaria. 1982. 'Population', in Dharma Kumar (ed.), *The Cambridge Economic History of India*, Hyderabad: Orient Longman, Vol 2, 463–532.

Watkins, S.C. 1993. 'If all we Knew about Women was What we Read in Demography, What Would we Know?' *Demography*, 30 (4): 551–7.

CHAPTER I

# *Introduction*

A great deal has been written on population and fertility by demographers, economists and, of late, sociologists and psychologists. Since the early 1960s there has been a spate of empirical studies on fertility determinants, differentials and change. Yet the problem of population growth continues to intrigue researchers. Fertility trends still pose major dilemmas for policy makers, administrators and others the world over, particularly in the Third World.

Fertility research has been dominated by demographers and economists. The demographic problem remained marginal to the central concern of classical sociological theories. Sociologists and social anthropologists have ventured into this area relatively recently. Population studies in general have received scant attention from sociologists, especially in India.

The present research attempts a holistic perspective on fertility behaviour through a monographic study of a village community. A holistic perspective here means an integrated view of the village community and its functioning, especially in relation to people's fertility. The aim is to understand fertility behaviour as an integral part of village society.

Stepping back for a moment, our understanding would benefit from an overview of the significant trends in the study of fertility. (For reviews of fertility studies, see Hawthorn 1970, UN 1973, Freedman 1975, 1979, Miro and Potter 1980, Caldwell *et al.* 1987.) The broad theoretical positions in fertility studies are examined here with a view to working out a conceptual framework for an understanding of fertility behaviour. Following Demeny (1981), past studies are classified by discipline and methodological approach. There are four prominent trends: macro-structural, micro-economic, psycho-social, and socio-economic.

Demeny classifies macro-structural and socio-economic studies under 'general socio-economic studies'. Within this broad category he then distinguishes between the macro- and micro-levels. I have, however, separated the two levels for as many reasons. First, macro-level studies have contributed largely to the advancement of the theory of demographic transition (one of the three important theories of population, the other two being Malthusian and Marxian). Secondly, my study refers frequently to micro-level studies. Hence, the need to deal with them separately.

The macro-structural perspective of 'demographic transition' is propounded by Thompson (1929), Notestein (1945), Kirk (1971), Repetto (1979) and Mauldin and Berelson (1978). It focusses on societies and regions as units of analysis, and shows that modernization and development lead to decline in fertility. It claims that rationality comes only with industrial and urban society, while traditional agrarian societies are essentially superstitious. Closely related to the macro-level studies are the micro-level socio-economic ones which focus on the household as the unit of analysis. Based largely on sample surveys, these are correlation and regression analyses of fertility in relation to social and economic variables, such as income, women's status, education and age at marriage.

These studies assume the dominance of social, structural and socio-economic factors in constraining fertility outcomes of passive or docile couples. Macro-structural and socio-economic theories in their analyses of fertility differentials are scarcely concerned with the purposes of human agents and their subjective orientations. The socio-economic circumstances are supposed to act upon couples with little regard for what they may feel or believe about them. In fact, most studies relate socio-economic variables directly to fertility without attempting to probe the numerous interlinkages between the two as though a given fertility configuration merely 'happens' to couples.

The micro-economic (also called 'human capital') theories analyse couples in reproductive ages as being at centre stage (Becker 1960, 1965, Lancaster 1966, Easterlin 1975). They explain fertility decision-making of a couple in terms of economic costs and benefits, applying the laws of consumer choice, of demand and supply, and of new home economics. Couples are regarded as rational consumers regulating their fertility in terms of costs and benefits with the purpose of maximizing statisfaction. They argue that a couple would desire a child as long as it has a utility function greater than its utility cost. They treat children as consumer durables. They do not, however, take into consideration the unacknowledged factors behind fertility often overlooking the fact that before having a child couples seldom calculate the economic implications of their behaviour.

The psycho-social theories differ sharply from the micro-economic approach (Pohlman 1969, Fawcett 1970, 1972, 1976, 1986, Arnold *et al.* 1975). They focus on couples in the reproductive age and emphasize non-economic values, such as satisfactions and utilities of children as perceived by couples. Fertility determinants are conceptualized in terms of beliefs, feelings and values related to childbearing preferences. The famous 'value-of-children' studies, and KAP (Knowledge, Attitude, and Practice) surveys of fertility and contraception belong to this category.

The micro economic and psycho-social studies view fertility behaviour as a result of factors that actors comprehend and control. In other words, couples on the basis of their knowledge and assessment tend to 'make hapen' a given fertility pattern. These studies over-emphasize the calculative knowledge of couples in deciding about their fertility while ignoring historical experiences and socio-economic conditions of the larger society in the context of which a given fertility behaviour occurs. In sharp contrast, macro-level studies remain silent about the day-to-day social activity of the reproductive agents.

Each of the above approaches emphasizes certain variables and ignores certain others. Overall, they focus either on the subjective orientations of actors or on the broad objective/structural features of the society circumscribing fertility behaviour. Although the four types of studies suffer from shortcomings, they have contributed immensely to the understanding of fertility.

### *Focus and Framework of the Present Study*

Here, the divide between the subjective and objective frame works is taken as the point of departure. Social practices are at the root of objective conditions and their perceptions. The premise of this study, taken from Giddens (1984), is that the existing *dualism* in the understanding of fertility behaviour should be reconceptualized as a *duality*—as two facets of a single phenomenon. Dualism means that objective conditions and people's perceptions are two independent phenomena, while duality means that they together constitute the medium as well as the outcome of recursive social practices. The important question in the duality of structure may be put as: Which processes make a couple incorporate and regenerate the overall fertility pattern in and through their own reproductive behaviour?

Drawn from Giddens' (1984: 1–34) concept of structuration, it seeks to relate the category of action and meaning to that of rules, resources and institutional framework. Fertility behaviour here is to be located neither in the experience of the individual actor nor in the existence of any form of societal totality, but in social practices occurring routinely. The various social practices associated with fertility are recursive—repetitive activities undertaken in a like manner day after day.

To see how fertility behaviour goes on recursively over time, the developmental process of the household is useful. Just as the household goes through a developmental process, the husband-wife couple also follow a socially expected and regulated 'fertility career'. How do various processes functioning in the life of a couple influence the developmental phases of their fertility career?

Relevant to our understanding is the knowledgeability of couples which is always present in recursive social practices associated with fertility behaviour. The emphasis is on what Giddens (1984: 41) calls active reflexive character of human conduct. Fertility is the outcome of knowledge—rational, evaluative, affectual or customary—which actors have about childbearing and rearing. In other words, people are not ignorant of what they do and whether a behaviour is expected of them or not. Continuity of practices presumes reflexivity, i.e., continuous monitoring of reproductive behaviour which couples perform and expect others to perform. Whatever couples know about their fertility behaviour is not restricted to reasons and rationalizations in their verbal expressions but is also embedded in what Giddens (1984) calls 'mutual knowledge'. This is traceable in people's behaviour carried on routinely in a taken-for-granted fashion. Mutual knowledge is not directly accessible in discursive terms. The domain of practical consciousness consists of all the things that couples know tacitly about how to 'go on' without being able to give them direct discursive expression.

What processes account for changes in fertility behaviour? In the event of such changes do couples have any control over their fertility behaviour and are they able to take liberties with the norm of socially-optimum number of children?

Thus the emphasis here is on analysis of fertility behaviour as grounded in the knowledgeable activities of couples who draw upon structures, including, among other things, rules and resources to carry on their social practices. The endeavour is to identify not only the socio-economic factors influencing fertility, but also the specific institutional mechanisms, i.e., customs, rituals, ceremonies, etc., through which these factors operate. The socio-economic factors and specific institutional mechanisms should be seen as an interrelated whole rather than as mutually exclusive and independent factors. I have attemped the study of fertility behaviour with this perspective in mind.

A major breakthrough in fertility studies in recent years are the intensive community studies. They belong to a much less common genre of research on fertility determinants and have yielded insights into the institutional setting of fertility behaviour. Some of these studies are: Caldwell (1976 and 1982) on the changing African family, Caldwell *et al.* (1984) on fertility in south India, White (1976) on labour absorpotion in rural Java, Parish and Whyte (1978) on social change in south China, and Cain *et al.* (1979) on patriarchal authority in rural Bangladesh and its implication for women's work and fertility. Another useful study, though not exactly on fertility behaviour, is Djurfeldt and Lindberg (1976) on health and health policies in a Tamil village in south India. The present work belongs to this genre.

Among human beings fertility refers to biological procreation. That is, the birth of a child as the result of a man impregnating a woman, and the latter delivering an infant after the gestation period. However, fertility can be measured by the number of children born to a woman without reference to the man who impregnated her. To avoid repetition, fertility is used here interchangeably with 'procreation' and 'reproduction', except that in certain contexts 'reproduction' is used in the social sense, as transmission of social and cultural characteristics.

This study deals with fertility behaviour of people in Mogra, a village in Jodhpur district of Rajasthan in north-western India (see Maps 1 and 2). Fertility behaviour refers to the processes of bearing and rearing children in the context of the household and the wider society. It covers the processes, including institutional mechanisms, leading directly or indirectly to childbirth and other demographic outcomes like child survival and mortality. People's concrete experiences impinging upon the process of child bearing and rearing in the village are seen as constituents of fertility behaviour. As Mckintosh states, fertility behaviour refers:

> . . . not merely to the bearing of children . . . but also to their care and socialization, and the maintenance of adult individuals through their lives, processes which create individuals to fit more or less into social structure of society and so ensure the continuation of that society in the next generation (1981: 9).

Besides childbearing, child care and provision of domestic and other services to adults also constitute the entire complex of fertility behaviour. Childbearing is, of course, the sole prerogative of women, but in the rearing and socialization of children husbands also have their socially-ordained responsibilities. Although mothers own the major share of these responsibilities, fathers also contribute in a number of ways. Moreover, childbearing and rearing are rarely the responsibility of a couple in isolation. The entire household, the family, the neighbourhood, and the network of relatives contribute in various ways. Thus, the mother in the centre and the other household members, relatives and neighbours around her in overlapping circles form the broad canvas of fertility behaviour in the village.

The major components of fertility behaviour, including the related institutional mechanisms, occupy most of this dissertation. Mortality and migration, the other two of the three processes of population, also receive attention but only in so far as they impinge

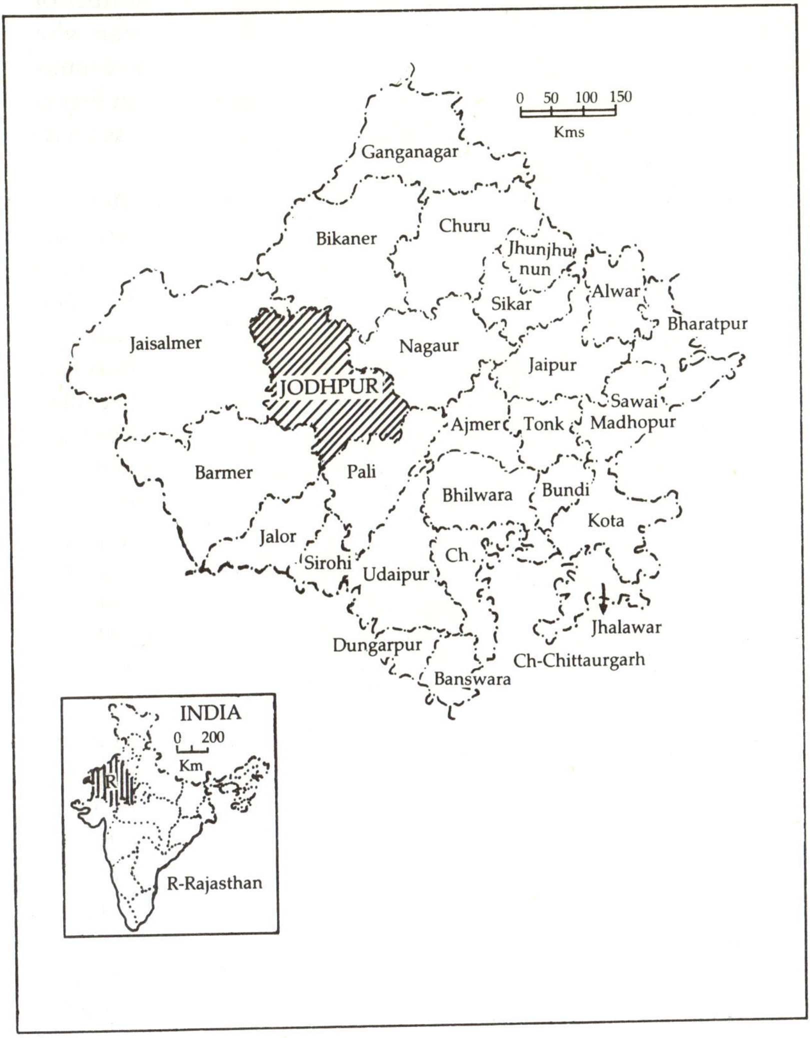


Map 1. Rajasthan and its Districts

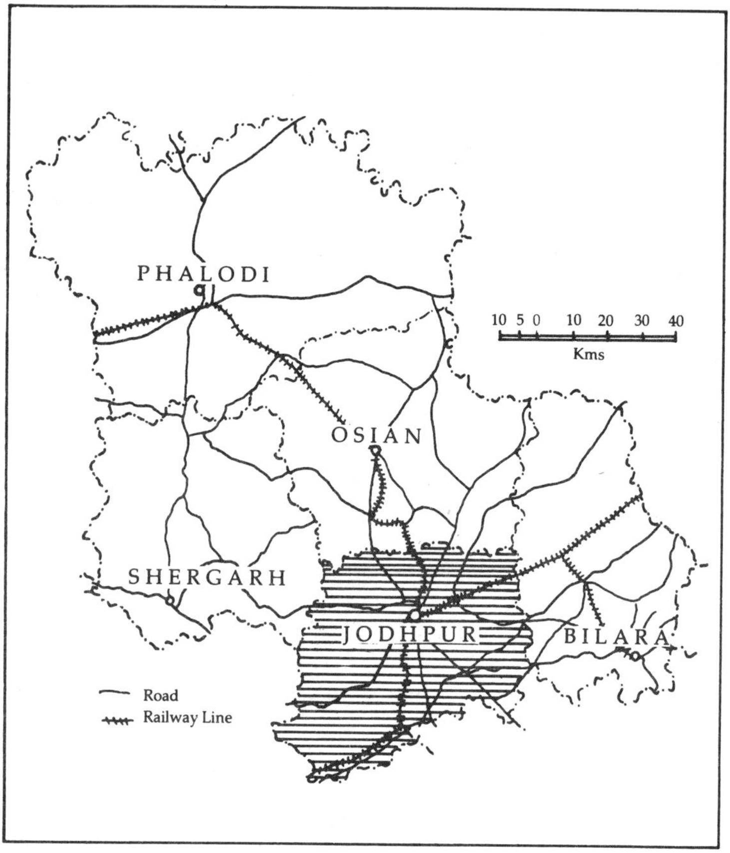


Map 2. Jodhpur and its Tehsils

upon and contribute to our understanding of fertility behaviour. The aim is to explore fertility behaviour as embedded in the framework of village society, and not simply to know fertility patterns, trends and estimates in statistical terms. While reproductive relations are at the centre of marriage and kinship relations they also circumscribe the operation of sexuality and fertility. The relations of marriage and kinship construct the context for bearing, caring and socializing children. Fertility behaviour permeates numerous dimensions of social, cultural and economic life. In short, the concern here is: How do various social processes, including institutional mechanisms, operate to enable couples to bear and rear children and continue to do so over time? Which processes bring about changes in fertility behaviour, and how?

### *Methodology*

This study is based mainly on the method of intensive fieldwork, identified by many as the anthropological method. This is a more fruitful manner of grasping the complexity of fertility behaviour, as advocated not only by anthropologists and sociologists but also by a few demographers (Rao 1974, Nag *et al.* 1978, Demeny 1981, Caldwell 1982, Handwerker 1986). They propose that in-depth studies using intensive interviews and participant observation are more meaningful than structured sample surveys, commonly employed to analyse fertility behaviour. The relationship between institutional setting and fertility can be worked out more adequately by intensive fieldwork. Caldwell *et al.* (1987) highlight the unique contribution of participant observation and the strength of prolonged personal contact with the field. While appreciating Schapera's (1955) study in Botswana, they state: We cannot understand what is happening to the birth rate among the Tswana unless we investigate the cultural setting of procreation (Caldwell *et al.* 1987: 28). They suggest that there is a need to go deeper into the dynamics of people's behaviour. Rao (1974) points out that an area of human behaviour as intimate as fertility behaviour cannot be understood by simply asking questions. Participant observation and case studies are helpful in providing access to this sensitive domain in human life.

Fertility research requires sensitivity to people's routine life.

Blanket judgements about them being ignorant or backward prevent understanding. One of the main reasons why fertility research—and fertility policy—have not been able to achieve a breakthrough is the ethnocentrism of researchers. Caldwell (1982: 86) points out how western notions about family, economy and reproductive decision-making are superimposed inaproppriately on non-western societies (see also Srinivas *et al.* 1979 for an elaboration ofhow urban intellectuals in India have little knowledge of, and respect and humility for, the rural, the poor, etc.). To consider a people under study as ignorant or irrational, is a colonial legacy in fieldwork. Giddens highlights how actors are knowledgeable about the norms of the society in which their actions take place: 'They know a great deal about the conditions and consequences of what they do in their day-to-day lives. All competent members of society are vastly skilled in the practical accomplishments of social activities' (1984: 26).

Since the purpose here is to understand the processes of fertility behaviour, rather than simply report on trends and patterns of fertility, meanings rather than frequencies of fertility assume greater significance. This is not to suggest, that it is futile to collect statistics and ask questions. But several questions may appear redundant if the researcher adopts the fieldwork method. Many questions may be considered worth laughing off. For instance, Caldwell (1982: 21) reports from his experience in African societies that it was ridiculous to ask how many children one desired to have. Similarly, when I asked my villagers about the contraceptives they used, I was laughed off, as my direct questions amused the elder, and embarassed the younger, women. It was only by living among them, and gossiping with them in groups and in the privacy of some corner in the house or the cattle shed, that I got to know several intimate details about contraception.

Dense descriptions of qualitative data support quantitative data (see Djurfeldt and Lindberg 1976: 9 for a discussion on a combination of this kind). The need to ask for explanations from people does not usually arise as expressive actions also transmit messages (see Leach 1976 for an elaborate discussion on this issue). As long as actions follow conventions, the message transmitted by one member is understood to be correct by other members of the society. A researcher can become familiar with and understand customary practices only through intensive fieldwork.

To obtain in-depth information, I studied the day-to-day life and conduct of the people. Instead of relying only on quantitative data, which is surely very useful, it was important to understand verbal and non-verbal modes of expression. Interpretation of expressions such as humour, sarcasm, applause, irony, facial movements and other linguistic and body gestures, provide important supportive data, otherwise absent in dry sample surveys. The above modes of expression, considered less important by conventional research in demography, enabled me to place the routine life of people in a context with both enabling and constraining features of interaction in Mogra. Caldwell (1982) states that small-scale, painstakingly thorough research on fertility has hardly been done by investigators with an in-depth knowledge of society. Mine is a modest attempt in this direction.

I spent over a year in 1984–5 living and working in Mogra. That year is my 'ethnographic present'. The present tense here refers to the time of my research. Occasional references to earlier and later visits have been stated as such. Past tense refers to the time prior to 1984–5. How I went about collecting data in Mogra is described in Appendix 1.

I shall discuss in Chapter 2 most of the quantitative data I collected in Mogra. It concerns 713 ever married women and their husbands. More quantitative data will be presented in Chapters 5 and 7. On the other hand, a considerable amount of qualitative data will be presented in the form of case studies in Chapters 3 to 7. The names of 34 men and 64 women concerning whom such data is presented are listed in Appendix 3. It is needless to add that I observed the behaviour of many more men and women during my fieldwork than those named here.

## *The Social Entity of Mogra*

Whether the Indian village is a social entity or not has been debated in sociological literature. But is it just an administrative and revenue unit? Or a mere architectural and demographic entity (Dumont and Pocock 1957)? Does it have a social and cultural identity (Srinivas 1975)? Or is it also a 'sociological reality' (Bailey 1959)?

Mahobia (1976) says that in Rajasthan, the smallest unit for land revenue and administration was called *gānv* in the 17th and 18th centuries, and that a person is also identified through his village. A village had ponds, wells, cultivable and pasture land, and borders called '*seenv*' or '*seem*'. Mogra has a housing settlement (*vasti*) and a surrounding land mass (*kaunkaḍ/hīm*). Both the *vasti* (also called *gānv* in certain contexts) and the *kaunkaḍ* constitute the physical setting of the geographical area of Mogra.

It is necessary to see if Mogra is a demographic unit. An ideal and typical demographic unit is one where birth, death, migration and marriage of all its people take place within its territorial boundary. In terms of the above notion, it is logically indefensible to consider Mogra as such. It is not possible to draw a boundary line around demographic phenomena, like birth, death, marriage and migration there. Many of these, of course, take place within the village, but many others involve people from outside also. Although a large number of its people are born in Mogra and are likely to live and die there, many others do not fall in this category. For instance, most wives migrate into Mogra and most daughters from Mogra go to other villages on marriage. Interdependence between Mogra and other areas is relevant not only for marital alliances and the relations ensuing from them, but also for births. A woman's first childbirth takes place in her natal home even if the child belongs to its father's village (Mogra). Emigrants and immigrants show Mogra's demographic interrelation with other places. We shall later discuss immigrants belonging to other villages and towns settled in Mogra, and vice versa. Nevertheless, Mogra does have a stable population of different age, sex and other demographic categories, that are enumerable by employing census procedures. Although Mogra may not be a unit encompassing all demographic features, it is a viable unit within which several critical demographic variables play their part.

Mogra, as mentioned earlier, is located in a semi-arid desert area in Jodhpur district, one of the 26 districts of Rajasthan state. Like almost one-half of this state, Jodhpur is situated between 75° and 73°15′ east longitudes and 26°10′ north latitude, at an altitude of 150 to 300 metres. It comprises five *tehsils*. Mogra is one of the 192 villages in Jodhpur *tehsil* (see Map 3). Local administration is

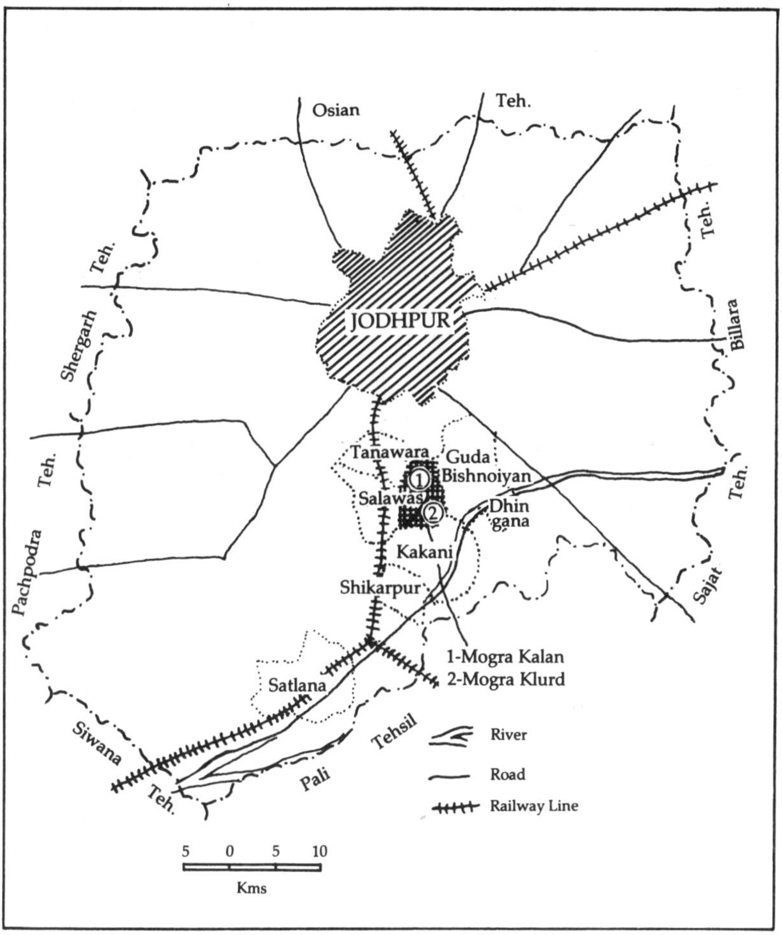


Map 3. Jodhpur Tehsil Mogra and its Neighbouring Villages

the jurisdiction of Luni panchayat *samiti*, one of the two committees that manage the affairs of the villages of Jodhpur *tehsil*. Most of Jodhpur district is a sandy plain dotted with hillocks. Mogra is 25 kilometres south of Jodhpur city and lies on the highway that connects the city to Pali, the headquarter town of the adjacent Pali district.

For several decades, the housing settlement of Mogra has been divided into two parts: Kalan and Khurd. They are on either side of the Jodhpur-Pali highway. Kalan is larger. The Census of India considers them as different villages. They had different patterns of land revenue until the abolition of *jagirs* in 1952. Kalan was a *khalsa* (ryotwari) and Khurd a *jagir* village. The *jagir* was held by members of the Charan caste. After 1952, it was converted, like many other *jagir* villages in the region, into a *khalsa* village. Nowadays, for all administrative purposes, there is a common *sarpanch* (head of the village panchayat) and *patwari* (revenue accountant) for the two parts of Mogra and one adjoining village. Practically and socially, Kalan and Khurd constitute one Mogra village and are regarded here as such.

Like a few other villages in the region, Mogra was electrified two years ago. There was no electricity in Mogra during my earlier fieldwork in 1980–1. The village pond and well were the only sources of water. Lately, the government has constructed a large water tank and bored a few tube wells in Mogra. The people of this area, including Mogra, have for long suffered from a water-borne disease caused by guinea worm called *vāḷo* though its incidence has declined considerably in recent years.

Usually, the houses of one caste are located near one another. Members of a caste reside adjacent to one another on the same *gali* (street) or, if their number is large, in a single *vah* (ward), a unit of a few streets adjacent to one another. If the population of a caste is small, more than one caste resides on the same street. A street or ward is named after the caste numerically dominant in it. For instance, there is Charan *vah*, Bhambi *vah*, jat *vah*, Raika *vah*, Brahmin *vah*, etc. While the members of a large caste, and sometimes those of a large patrilineage within a caste, reside adjacent to one another, the minor castes do not have their own wards or even streets. They live on streets with mixed population.

For instance, a few Saad, Saami, Kumbar and Jat houses are on one street.

The untouchable castes reside on the outskirts of the village settlement, while the central part is occupied by the higher castes. However, this caste-based settlement pattern has been changing in recent years. The settlement is spreading beyond the erstwhile untouchable caste streets on the outskirts.

There are six temples (*mindar*) and several smaller shrines (*thān*) in Mogra. Three of the temples are located in the central settlement, with either Brahmin and mendicant caste houses close to them. One temple was being constructed during my stay. Of the remaining two temples, one is located near the village well and the other, called Bhakri, on a hillock about 2 kilometres from Mogra.

There are three schools. One of them is a middle school. The other two are primary schools, of which one is exclusively for girls. One was set up in 1973, and the other, towards the end of my fieldwork in 1985. The middle school is the oldest. Its primary section was started in 1954, and upgraded in 1972. Schooling of children is, however, not a priority for parents in Mogra. Sending girls to school is rarer than sending boys. Of the 360 students enrolled in the middle school, only 24 are girls. In one of the primary schools there are 47 boys and 23 girls. In the exclusively girls' primary school, 100 girls are registered but only about 30 actually attend it.

Like other villages in the region, there are internal differences in Mogra along caste, class and other lines. Despite caste differentiation, the castes in the village interact with each other and there are certain symbols of the village as a collectivity. These include the village settlement (*vasti*), the *hīm* (agricultural land), the catchment area (*oraṇ*), the grazing ground (*gocher*), the main entrance to the village settlement (*phaḷo*), the pond, the well, fairs and festivals, Bhakri (the Shiva temple), shrines and shamans, and the crematorium. While the members of Mogra may either visit or live in a neighbouring village, the identity of most of the members with their 'motherland' (*jalam bhom*), the village, is quite strong. The immigrants, of course, do not consider it their 'motherland'. The same holds true for women from other villages married into Mogra, during the initial phase of their married life. They come to take it as their village gradually. Besides, people have their houses and land and other means of livelihood in the village. Even when they find employment outside Mogra, most of their family and social life is spent in the village.

Certain ritual and symbolic acts give the *phaḷo* its social existence. Members of all castes perform certain rituals at the *phaḷo* on the occasions of wedding and cremation. When a boy's wedding procession leaves the village, it halts at the *phaḷo* for performing a ritual to the four directions. When such a procession from another village arrives at the *phaḷo*, the bride's relatives go to receive it, and after the wedding, they see the procession off at the *phaḷo*. Here the bride's face is washed ceremonially and offerings are made in the four directions. Similarly, the groom's procession on its return with the bride halts at the *phaḷo* before proceeding to the groom's house. Upon an adult's death the bier is lowered at the *phaḷo* to pay last homage to the village before proceeding to the crematorium. If a person dies outside the village, the dead body is first brought to the village. Similarly an outsider (not belonging to the village) is usually not cremated at the village crematorium. The body is instead taken to its own village. In addition, the *phaḷo* symbolizes security inside and insecurity outside. Once inside the *phaḷo*, a person is safe from all insecurities. It is also believed that a person is possessed by demons and devils only beyond the *phaḷo*, not within the village settlement. Whenever one is possessed, exorcists drive away the demons beyond the *phaḷo*.

The village as a collectivity organizes fairs on auspicious days, and its members participate in the major Hindu festivals. As mentioned earlier, several temples and shrines belong to the village. The village members are obliged to pay some amount in cash or kind to the priests of these temples. The untouchables, of course, participate in temple rituals from a distance. Although several shrines and shamans are visited by people from outside, these are believed to belong to Mogra. The newely-weds are obliged to pay homage to the village shrines and temples. The Shiva temple called Bhakri is situated in the village *hīm*. A majority of the people believe the Bhākri to be a protection against epidemics, famines, etc. It is believed to bring peace and well-being to the people of Mogra. Last but not least, the Bhangi (scavenger) belongs to the village. He is paid for his work at a piece-rate, and gets in addition occasional obligatory gifts and other payments.

For over seven decades, each household in Mogra Khurd has sent meals for the Bhakri priest every morning by turn. People of Mogra Kalan also offer meals, grains, etc., but they do not observe the morning meal obligation. Political candidates begin their campaigns by first offering worship at the Bhakri temple.

The pond, the well, the *gocher* and the *oraṇ* belonging to the village community provide several amenities to the villagers. Their own needs of water and fuel, and their cattle's requirements of water and grazing are fulfilled by these common resources. People participate not only in their regular use but also in their protection and maintenance. For instance, in summer months before the onset of monsoons a few women and girls desilt the village pond in the early morning hours.

The village exists in the consciousness of its people as an anchorage and social entity. They are clear that they belong to Mogra. Those girls going as brides to other villages are called 'Mogra's daughters' (*Mogra ree bēti*). Brides coming into Mogra are called 'Mogra's brides' (*Mogra ree voo*). A person's identification in this region includes at least three indicators: (1) one's name and father's name, (2) caste, and (3) village. The sense of belonging and the relationships based on face-to-face interaction in the village are reflected in the manner in which people address one another by fictional kinship terms. It is common for people of the same age group to address each other by their personal names. The younger ones are also similarly addressed. Suffixes such as brother (*bhāi*) or sister (*bāi/bein*) for slightly senior persons are used with their names, and persons belonging to one's parental generation are called *kāka* and *kāki* (father's younger brother and his wife respectively). The aged are addressed as *bapu* (grandfather and his equivalent) and *maa* (grandmother or equivalent). This practice cuts across caste groups. An important link binding village members together as members of the community is the wedding feast. Similarly, on the third day of an adult member's death, the entire village participates in the mourning. All the village residents are invited to the mortuary feast *gānv ghātḍi*. People in the village share with its emigrants a common identity. It is not uncommon for a person from Mogra to visit an emigrant non-kin settled in a town or city and be greeted with warmth and treated with tea, and at times even with meals. Mogra is indeed a social and cultural entity with a consciousness of kind, i.e., people have a feeling of belonging, a certain sense of mutual responsibility.

### *The Selection of Mogra*

One reason for choosing Mogra was the lack of any intensive sociological study of villages in western Rajasthan. There are a few surveys (Bose and Malhotra 1964; Bose and Jodha 1965) of agriculture, sheep raising, etc. But these are no substitute for a fieldwork-based full-length sociological study.

Other considerations behind my choice of Mogra were its proximity to Jodhpur city and the location of its housing settlement on the highway. An added advantage was the location of two houses, on either side of the road at Mogra's bus stop, whose members were ever ready to accompany me at odd hours to the village settlement which being at a distance from the road posed problems of transport and of personal security, especially when people knew that a female researcher was working all alone.

Mogra also happens to be my father's ancestral village. He migrated and settled in Jodhpur city about five decades ago. As people in Mogra saw me in terms of their cordial relations with him, I anticipated little problem in having access to and building rapport with the people. The image of a 'daughter of Mogra', as well as some rapport-building skills proved helpful. I am well-versed in the local dialect, and therefore did not take long to learn the local proverbs and idioms. The study of Mogra may thus be considered as study of my own society, but it is also important to note that it is not easy to define one's society. There are social, cultural and dialectual variations within a region/state and even a district, which make one feel a stranger in one's own society in more ways than one (Srinivas *et al.* 1979).

Another major reason for selecting Mogra was that I knew it from two earlier field experiences. In 1980 I had conducted a small study on the fertility behaviour of Patel caste women in Mogra. It appeared as an article in 1982. The second fieldwork was in 1981—a village census for my M. Phil. dissertation. By the time I began fieldwork for this study in mid-1984, I had acquired enough familiarity with the village. I completed my fieldwork by end-1985. I stayed in the village intermittently till the first quarter of 1985 and continuously thereafter for the rest of the year. As I was visiting the village two or three times a year since 1980, I could afford to be away for short intervals during the first quarter of 1985 to resume teaching in Delhi and reflect on my work.

I knew that some persons in Mogra had access to city life and some formal education in and outside the village. They had urban occupations and availed of modern health care in the village as well as in the city. Mogra thus offered itself as a rural society having important linkages with the city. It thus revealed a scenario of social continuity as well as of change whose impact on people's fertility behaviour was worth studying.

An in-depth study of as intimate a subject as human fertility requires prolonged participant observation. Since I had maintained ties with Mogra as a researcher, I felt assured that it would be advantageous to work in a village I was familiar with.

### *Demographic Profile of Mogra*

Mogra is a large village. Only 13 of the 192 villages in the Jodhpur *tehsil* are larger than Mogra Kalan and Khurd put together. Two of them, Salawas and Gura Bishnoiya, are situated within a distance of about 3 kilometres.

Mogra has 2,748 persons living in 410 households, belonging to 23 castes. Of them 1,413 (51.41%) are men and 1,335 (48.59%) women. (See Table 1.1 for village population by sex and age) The sex ratio in Mogra is more favourable to women than that in Rajasthan or the country as a whole. It was 944 in Mogra, 921 in Rajasthan, and 935 in India in 1981 (Census of India 1981a). In this respect, Mogra is an atypical village. Only a comparative study can reveal why this is so.

The sex ratio varies with age groups. In the above 56 age group, it is favourable to women. In the 46–60 years age group it is 1,111. A larger proportion of women is found in the above 60 age group: 44 men, 57 women. But the sex ratio in the other age groups is

TABLE 1.1 *Distribution of population by sex and age*

| Age group (in years) | POPULATION Male | (%) | Female | (%) | Total | (%) | Sex ratio |
|---|---|---|---|---|---|---|---|
| 0–5 | 251 | (17.76) | 252 | (18.87) | 503 | (18.30) | 1,003 |
| 6–10 | 227 | (16.06) | 200 | (14.98) | 427 | (15.53) | 881 |
| 11–15 | 169 | (11.96) | 151 | (11.31) | 320 | (11.64) | 893 |
| 16–20 | 155 | (10.96) | 127 | ( 9.51) | 282 | (10.26) | 819 |
| 21–25 | 119 | (8.42) | 111 | (8.31) | 230 | (8.36) | 932 |
| 26–30 | 121 | (8.56) | 123 | (9.21) | 244 | (8.87) | 1,016 |
| 31–35 | 75 | (5.30) | 65 | (4.86) | 140 | (5.09) | 866 |
| 36–40 | 76 | (5.37) | 77 | (5.76) | 153 | (5.56) | 987 |
| 41–45 | 57 | (4.03) | 49 | (3.67) | 106 | (3.85) | 859 |
| 46–50 | 50 | (3.53) | 49 | (3.67) | 99 | (3.60) | 980 |
| 51–55 | 31 | (2.19) | 26 | (1.94) | 57 | (2.07) | 838 |
| 56–60 | 37 | (2.61) | 48 | (3.59) | 85 | (3.09) | 1,297 |
| 61 and above | 44 | (3.11) | 57 | (4.26) | 101 | (3.67) | 1,295 |
| Total | 1,413 | (100) | 1,335 | (100) | 2,748 | (100) | 944 |

much below the national and state averages. It does not favour women before the age of 45. In age groups 15–30 and 31–45, it is 913 and 918 respectively. Ruzicka (1984) rightly observes that the anomaly of longer life expectation of males than of females obtains in India and other countries of the subcontinent. It results from higher age-specific female mortality at most ages under 50.

These are considerable number of old people in the village. The oldest man and woman are aged 95 and 90 respectively. It is possible for a young boy to find his father's father living at the time of his marriage. As marriages occur at an early age, people become grandparents around 40 years of age. People are considered especially lucky if they survive to see their son's son's children.

Despite checks and counter questions to arrive at an approximate age of the population during my census in 1984, not all age figures are accurate. In the village culture, certain digits are preferred when people measure time in terms of their age, events in the calendar, history of the village, or the individual's biographical trajectory. The sequence of time is grasped invariably with a digital preference for five and multiples and for certain even numbers such as 'two' and 'eight'. People state their age in terms of a pair of numerals, such as 8–10, 20–22, 24–25 and so on. A low rate of literacy as well as a lack of need to either recall or write dates of birth, partly explain people's indifference to exact numerals. Sometimes a social position (as for example, married, unmarried, or having grandchildren) influences the estimation of age. Ages of unmarried girls of marriageable age are usually under-reported and those of adolescent married girls over-stated. After having a few children or after the marriage of their children, older people tend to exaggerate their age.

Some people are domiciled in Mogra but reside outside the village. Of these, some have government jobs, while others are engaged in business. Most of them live in various districts of Rajasthan and a few in other states. All these people have set up households at their places of work. They maintain a variety of links with the village, by having land, houses and relatives in the village. But the duration and frequency of visits vary from individual to individual. They have, as it were, one foot in the village and the other outside it. Following Shah (1973), the emigrants may be classified as 'independent' and 'linked'. Independent emigrants are those who have independent or separate houses, and live in these houses when they visit the village. Linked emigrants are those who do not have separate houses of their own, and reside in the houses of their parents, brothers, sons, and such other close relatives when they come to the village. Those who commute to town for work and return to the village every day are not emigrants. There are also a few who have renounced the world for the sake of religion and move from place to place. These I call 'vagrants'.

Not all emigrants are regarded here as constituting the village population. Vagrants and those independent emigrants who did not visit the village for more than a year during my fieldwork, are excluded. One of the reasons being my inability to meet and obtain data from them. On the other hand, three households of immigrants, i.e., outsiders residing in Mogra for a few years, are included as constituting the village population. One of them is a school teacher belonging to a village in another tehsil in Jodhpur district. He has been living in Mogra with his wife and son for about 14 years. The second is constituted of a doctor, his wife (a teacher) their two daughters and a son. They have been living in Mogra for over two years. The third is a single-member household of a female nurse employed in the village dispensary. She has been living in Mogra for over five years. All the three households play an active role in the social life of the village. Other outsiders employed in Mogra, who usually commute, and occasionally live in the village for a few months, are not included in the village census. Nevertheless, their interaction with people in Mogra is discussed.

### *Castes in Mogra*

Caste is an important aspect of the social structure of Mogra as of any village in India. Indeed it would be nearly impossible to discuss any major aspect of village life in India without relating it to its constituent castes. The term caste is used here to connote *jati*, the smallest endogamous group with a certain status in the ritual hierarchy of Hindu society. In Mogra and the neighbouring villages, the term *jati* (or *jat*, to be more specific) is used to mean caste.

The caste groups in the village are part of horizontal caste units. The population of a caste is spread over a certain region or even all over India. It is represented in different villages and even in towns in different numbers and proportions. The inter-village caste organization is called *chautalo* in the region around Mogra. It is an indicator of a caste's regional solidarity. Its territorial extent differs from caste to caste.

Almost the entire population of Mogra is Hindu, except one Bhil, and three Muslim Teli, households. The Bhil and Teli behave more or less like caste groups. Srinivas (1965: 6) points out that although by Islamic dogma Muslims do not have a caste system, in actual practice, Indian Muslims are divided into caste-like groups. This is also true of Mogra. Muslims belong to the Teli (oil presser) caste. The Bhil are, truly speaking, a scheduled tribe, and do not come under the fold of the Hindu caste system. But the Bhils in Mogra are considered more or less untouchable. Although hypergamous marriages between Bhil and Rajput and consequently the enhanced status of Bhils have been reported (see Chauhan 1967: 89–90 and Shah and Desai 1988: 16), the purpose here is to see the status of the Bhils in relation to other castes in Mogra. None of the higher caste members accept food or water from the Bhil and Teli in Mogra, though they visit their homes, which they do not do with the untouchable castes.

The 23 castes in Mogra differ from one another in population and number of households (see Table 1.2 for households and population by caste in Mogra). Each caste has a ritual status in the caste hierarchy. Srinivas (1955) states that though there are ranked differences of castes, it is difficult to determine even the approximate place of each in the hierarchical system. Any hierarchical

TABLE 1.2 *Distribution of village households and population by caste*

| *Caste* | *Traditional calling* | *Number of households* | % | *Population* | % |
|---|---|---|---|---|---|
| Bania | Trader | 1 | (00.2) | 5 | (00.18) |
| Bhambi (Meghwal) | Leather worker | 43 | (10.4) | 237 | (08.62) |
| Bhangi | Scavenger | 1 | (00.2) | 6 | (00.21) |
| Bhil | Guard | 1 | (00.2) | 5 | (00.18) |
| Brahmin | Priest | 16 | (03.9) | 103 | (03.74) |
| Charan | Bard/landlord | 26 | (06.3) | 124 | (04.51) |
| Darjee | Tailor | 8 | (01.9) | 39 | (01.41) |
| Daroga | Servant of Rajput | 2 | (00.48) | 5 | (00.18) |
| Dholi | Drummer | 2 | (00.48) | 15 | (00.54) |
| Jat | Cultivator | 21 | (05.21) | 130 | (04.73) |
| Kareegar (Suthar) | Carpenter | 15 | (03.65) | 88 | (03.20) |
| Kumbar | Potter | 6 | (01.40) | 50 | (01.81) |
| Lawar | Blacksmith | 4 | (00.90) | 28 | (01.01) |
| Nai | Barber | 8 | (01.90) | 38 | (01.38) |
| Patel | Cultivator | 163 | (39.7) | 1,265 | (46.00) |
| Raika | Shepherd | 37 | (09.0) | 229 | (08.33) |
| Rajput | Ruler/warrior | 1 | (00.2) | 6 | (00.21) |
| Saad | Mendicant/priest (Vaishnavite) | 17 | (04.1) | 142 | (05.16) |
| Saami | Mendicant/priest (Shaivite) | 3 | (00.7) | 18 | (00.65) |
| Sargara | Menial servant | 29 | (07.0) | 177 | (06.44) |
| Sonar | Goldsmith | 2 | (00.48) | 17 | (00.61) |
| Teli | Oil presser | 3 | (00.7) | 18 | (00.65) |
| Vishnoi | Cultivator | 1 | (00.2) | 3 | (00.10) |
| Total | | 410 | (100.00) | 2,748 | (100.00) |

list is tentative and open to argument. However, the caste order is not inchoate. People have been able to carry on their functions without any major confusion about it. To comprehend it, Srinivas distinguishes between ritual and secular hierarchy of castes, and between a hierarchy as conceptualized by people and as it exists in actual behaviour, with economic, political and westernization factors playing an important part.

Although the primary purpose here is to understand fertility behaviour and not a detailed analysis of caste, some understanding of caste dynamics is essential to analyse reproductive behaviour in the village. Indeed caste has been frequently correlated with fertility in demographic studies in India. For a meaningful analysis of the relationship between the two in Mogra, I shall classify the castes into four categories on the basis of diet, occupation, customs and the nature of interaction among them.

In terms of diet, occupation and customs, the castes in Mogra are neither identical nor entirely dissimilar. Certain castes are more similar to one another than with certain others. These overall similarities and differences help us classify them into four categories: upper, upper-middle, lower-middle, and lower (see Table 1.3). This classification is similar to that done by K. L. Sharma (1974) for six villages in Rajasthan (cf. also Chauhan 1967 and Atal 1968).

We have to see the traditional calling, diet, and customs of marriage and kinship of the castes against the backdrop of the purity-pollution criterion. The Brahmin's traditional calling of priesthood is ranked highest in the ritual order, followed by those of the ruler/warrior (Rajput), the bard (Charan), and the trader (Bania). Below this category are the upper-middle castes, largely

TABLE 1.3 *Caste categories in Mogra*

| *Category* | *Castes* |
|---|---|
| Upper | Brahmin, Bania, Charan, Rajput |
| Upper-middle | Jat, Patel, Raika, Vishnoi |
| Lower-middle | Darjee, Daroga, Kareegar (Suthar), Kumbar, Lawar, Nai, Saad, Saami, Sonar |
| Lower | Bhambi, Bhangi, Bhil, Dholi, Sargara, Teli |

peasants (Jat, Patel, and Vishnoi) with agriculture as their sole traditional calling, and the semi-nomadic shepherds (Raika). Despite the difference of traditional calling, the Raika enjoy a ritual status similar to that of the Jat, Patel and Vishnoi. The lower-middle category includes artisan castes, mendicants, and Daroga (servants exclusively of rulers). Daroga and Nai perform certain tasks that are more polluting than those of Blacksmiths (Lawar) and Potters (Kumbar). A ritual bath after certain polluting tasks restores ritual purity to the Daroga and Nai—a privilege not available to the lower castes. The lower castes include the untouchables, namely, Bhambi (leather worker), Bhangi (scavenger and remover of dead cattle), and Sargara (menial servant on farms and cattlesheds, runner of errands, attender at births, and drummer for lower castes). The Bhambi and Sargara are ritually more polluting than others in this category, namely, Dholi (drummer), Bhil (a scheduled tribe) and Teli (Muslim oil-presser). The latter three are nearly untouchable. The Teli is so more for being a Muslim than for his calling of oil pressing.

With a few exceptions, the larger the number of castes serving a caste, the higher its ritual status. Castes not served by a caste but serving it instead have a lower status. The service-giving castes generally accept food from service-receiving ones. The nature of services provided also matters for a caste's status. The rituals performed by the Brahmin have high social and religious status, and despite his priestly services in temples and in households of all the upper, upper-middle and lower-middle castes, his status remains the highest. Although the Brahmin performs rituals for other castes, he accepts, not food but only *pētiyo* (victuals) from them.

The durable relation between the food-producing castes and the castes supplying them with goods and services is typical of *jajmani* relations (Wiser 1936). The upper-middle and upper castes, barring the Brahmin, offer little ritual services to other castes. The lower-middle castes, comprising mainly artisans, serve all except the lower castes on certain ritual occasions. As already mentioned, the services of Nai and Daroga are not offered to the lower castes, as their services are more prone to defilement than those of the Carpenter, the Blacksmith, etc. However, even a Carpenter or a Potter may not always provide goods/services to the lower castes, especially on ritual occasions. The Mendicants do not accept alms from the lower castes nor does the Dholi serve them. The latter have their own priests, barbers and drummers. (See Pocock 1962 for an analysis of *jajmani* relations, distinguishing between castes offering services and castes offering goods, and between ceremonial and ritual services, to highlight the difference between open and closed specializations of various castes).

Vegetarianism and teetotalism are ranked as superior attributes of a caste. By this criterion most of the vegetarian castes enjoy a high rank while the non-vegetarian castes belong to the lower category, except Charan and Rajput who belong to the highest category, despite being non-vegetarian and non-teetotaler. The non-vegetarianism of Charan and Rajput has, however, one connotation while that of the lower castes has another. The Bhambi, Bhangi and Sargara eat carrion, which Charan and Rajput do not. True to their martial tradition, they occasionally hunt animals and birds for food. Ritual defilement through alcohol and non-vegetarian food among the Charan and Rajput is considered temporary as against permanent ritual defilement of the untouchables.

Customs of marriage and kinship are more important than vegetarianism and teetotalism for caste ranking. Mogra is a monogamous and patrivirilocal society. Girls move out of the natal, and into the conjugal home on marriage. Parents are keen to marry their daughters around puberty, though not all marriages conform. As age at marriage is crucially linked to the status of women, and fertility in demographic studies, it is important to make a distinction between wedding and marriage. A wedding is a ritual and festive ceremony whereas marriage is cohabitation. A wedding is called *vīva* or *pannāvṇo*, while marriage is called *muklāwo, ano* (to bring, to come), *hāvarē mēlno* (to send to the conjugal home), or *kānchaḷi dēṇo* (made to wear a blouse meant for a married women), which is the jural sanction of marriage. When a girl leaves the parental home for the conjugal she is made to wear a special blouse called *kānchaḷi* with strings tied at the back. The bigger blouse covering her torso (the entire upper part) is discarded for good. The married woman then wears the *kānchaḷi* all her life. Upon widowhood she wears a dull coloured simple version.

The distinction between *vīva* and *muklāwo* is relevant for caste ranking. A daughter's wedding among the upper castes coincides with her marriage, while among the remaining three categories of castes such coincidence is not necessary. Daughters among the latter are wedded at an early age, i.e., they practise child-wedding. The girl's age at wedding can be any time from birth to about 18 years. Along with child-wedding they practise the institution of collective wedding of sisters when all the unwed daughters of a household are wedded together at the same time. Two brothers may occasionally come together and arrange the wedding of their unwed daughters (that is, classificatory sisters and/or daughters of a patriline) collectively at the same time. A group of sisters may be wedded along with their father's sisters if the latter happen to remain unmarried.

Such weddings enable households to economize on expenses, so much so, that if the groom's party is reluctant to participate in such a wedding, it is not only criticized severely for not bothering about the bride's father's expenses, but may risk breaking the betrothal. Collective weddings take place on two occasions: either when the eldest daughter reaches puberty and is to be married off, or when a mortuary feast is organized on the eleventh or twelfth day of an elderly parent's or grandparent's death.[1] However, each wedded daughter is sent to her conjugal household (for *muklāwo*) only at puberty, around the age of 15.

The norm is for the bride to be younger than her groom. The upper castes follow the norm more closely than do other castes. Among the former the age difference tends to be about 5–10 years, while among the other three caste categories it tends to vary, ranging from zero to several years. Among them, it is not difficult to find couples of equal age, and sometimes brides older than the groom. During the census, I encountered such cases. The respondents, their husbands and other household members how ever were reluctant to concede the fact that the wife was older and suggested that I make the bride seem younger as 'it does not "look good"

[1] The symbolism of the concurrence of wedding and mortuary feasts is not discussed here.

(when compared with upper caste customs) to write the wife as older than the husband'.

The upper castes pay susbstantial dowries and incur many other expenses on their daughters' weddings. On the other hand, the other three categories practise the custom of giving bride price for marrying their sons. In an attempt to Sanskritize, and at times to get an educated and employed groom for a daughter, an upper-middle or lower-middle caste family may not only waive the bride price but may also give some dowry. The attempt to Sanskritize is obvious among the upper-middle and lower-middle castes, who have nearly abandoned the custom of bride price. Nevertheless, the poorer among the upper-middle and lower-middle category take bride price for marrying their daughters, albeit clandestinely. Bride price is more openly prevalent among the lower castes. But one common feature among all castes is the giving of many customary gifts to sisters and daughters throughout their lifetime.

Barring the upper castes, the rest practise marriage by exchange (*hāto*), in which usually two men exchange their daughters so that each obtains a wife for his son. If a man has no daughter to offer in exchange for a daughter-in-law, he may offer his unmarried sister or his brother's unmarried daughter in exchange. Exchange marriage is practised only by those castes that have the institution of bride price. The *hāto* obviates the need for bride price and cancels out other obligatory prestations. The *hāto* is often expressed as *roti hātē roti* (literally, bread for bread). Nevertheless, *hāto* is generally not considered an ideal practice. Both bride price and *hāto* violate the Sanskritic ideology of *kanya dān* (gift of the virgin girl). However, the most common reason against *hāto* is that the relations ensuing from it are complicated and engender constant heartburning in the two households in the present and the next generation. *Hāto* is less common among the lower-middle castes than the upper-middle and lower castes.

Divorce is not customarily permitted among the upper castes. Among the rest, it is, in extreme cases. But the occasion arises only after a fairly protracted period of separation and after several efforts by kin and affines at patching up. If the issue is not solved, the final settlement of divorce occurs only with the intervention of the council of the *chautaḷo*. The caste elders (*panchas*) convey their judgement on formal divorce as well as on the punishment to be meted out to the natal families of either or both the concerned individuals. Their decision is called *pheslo* (literally, verdict). Both divorce and the *pancha's* verdict on it are so rare that there is no local term for divorce. It is simply said that the husband has driven his wife out (*kād di*) or *chhoḍe di* (left out).

Among the upper castes, expulsion spells doom for the wife. Her only place after marriage is her husband's home. She is unwanted in her parental home, and ceases to be a welcome guest there. She belongs to no one upon expulsion. She may be permitted prolonged residence at her parental home upon widowhood but rarely upon expulsion. She is then left to the mercy of her husband's agnates and his parents, who may allow her to stay on a plot of the household land. Only in extreme conditions, when she has no shelter in the conjugal household and is on the verge of destitution, does her natal household allow her to reside with them. She gets little regular support and has to survive on whatever she can manage to get from her natal or conjugal kin. The only upper caste deserted woman in Mogra, a Charan, was forced in the absence of any support, to give up *purdo* and move out to work on leased land for the sake of survival of self and children.

Expulsion among the upper-middle, lower-middle and lower castes does not spell as severe a doom for the woman. Nevertheless, it is a loss of status, and leaves a stigma on her. Unlike the upper castes, a man of the other castes cannot expel his wife easily. Marrying another woman once the first marriage is dissolved is not easy either. Unless a woman is unchaste she is rarely expelled. In case she is, without any convincing charge, her natal kin can protest before the caste council, and solicit their penalty for the offending man and his family. Arranging a second wife involves a great deal of expenditure for the man by way of high bride price and jewellery. The expelled woman usually reverts to her natal household, which arranges her remarriage (*nāta*). Divorce, although possible by both sexes among the three lower castes, is very rare. Divorce initiated by a woman is rarer. Although expulsion and divorce are more frequent among the lower castes, they are certainly not common.

Remarriage (*nāta*) of a widow or a divorced woman is an important institution distinguishing some castes from others. The upper castes do not permit it, while the other three categories do (cf. Atal 1968 for a similar situation in a southern Rajasthan village). *Nāta* is arranged invariably by the woman's natal relatives. It is linked to the institution of child-wedding. All except the upper castes practise both child-wedding and *nāta*. Among them a wedded daughter can be widowed after or prior to *muklāwo*. The *nāta* of a virgin-widow, one who has not undergone *muklāwo* despite being wedded (*pannāoḍi*), is known as *kanwāra* (unmarried virgin) *nāta*. Death of a prospective husband before *muklāwo* does not lead to loss of her virginity. Remarriage of a widow who has undergone *muklāwo* is called *nāta* with no adjective prefixed. Although *nāta* is permitted among all but the upper castes, women who become widows after having a few surviving children, particularly one son, rarely remarry (cf. Srinivas 1952 for a similar practice among the Coorgs). Among the upper-middle castes, in recent years, a few young widows with at least one child (a son or a daughter) have refused to remarry in an attempt to emulate the upper castes. In other words, the institution of *nāta* is on the decline, especially among the upper-middle and lower-middle castes—a marked indicator of their Sanskritization.

Remarriage does not have any of these preconditions for a man. He can remarry several women one after another upon widowerhood. His remarriage is not termed *nāta* unless he marries a widow or a deserted/divorced woman (possible only among the upper-middle, lower-middle and lower castes).

Sons are regarded as heirs to family property and status. Since the son perpetuates the patriline, his birth is considered essential. If no son is born, there are customary norms for dealing with such exceptions. In the absence of a son, it is considered ideal to adopt one. The adopted son gets legal heirship and associated rights and obligations. He legally belongs to his adopted father's family and lineage. It is ideal for a man to adopt his brother's, or another near agnate's, son. The upper castes maintain their distinct identity by meeting the ideal. The castes of the upper- and lower-middle category are fairly close to the ideal, while the lower castes are most liberal and rarely attach much value to the ideal. The adoptee parents in all except the upper castes consider cordiality of their relationship more important than agnatic ties while choosing a son for adoption.

In addition to adoption, the institution of *ghar jamāi* (literally, son-in-law in the house) is prevalent among the upper-middle, lower-middle, and lower castes. It helps maintain continuity of the family line and assures care to the aged. The *ghar jamāi* lives with his real or prospective wife in her natal home. He is brought in usually around the age of 10. He assists the elders in his prospective wife's household in agricultural and other tasks. Eventually he is formally married to a daughter in the household. The newly-wed couple continue to live there, unlike most other couples taking up patrivirilocal residence. The *ghar jamāi* becomes the jural heir of family property and status and fulfils all obligations expected of a son. Thus the upper-middle, lower-middle and lower castes adopt a son only when there is no surviving child in the family. If there is a daughter, they prefer to bring in a *ghar jamāi* rather than marry the daughter out and adopt a son as do the upper castes. The status of the daughter, in this respect, is higher among the latter three caste categories than among the upper castes. The incidence of *ghar jamāi* is more common among the upper-middle castes than among the lower-middle and lower castes.

Another striking difference between the castes concerns the ritual mortuary feast on the twelfth day of the father's and the eleventh day of the mother's death. This feast is of two kinds. One is a large-scale feast called *nyāt*, which goes on for three days, and to which all members of one's caste residing in the villages of the *chautāḷo* are invited. Another is a one-day feast called *gānv ghātḍi* (literally, porridge for the village) to which are invited all the village residents and the host's relatives residing outside the village. The village and caste elders (*panchās*) from the *chautāḷo* see to it that the feasts are organized upon the death of every elderly person, although the *panchās*' pressure, of late, is on the decline (see Atal 1968: 103 for a few cases dealing with the dynamics of decision-making for mortuary feasts). The mortuary feast is organized on a grand scale by the upper-middle castes. For both *nyāt* and *ghātḍi* feasts, they invite every resident of the village from all castes, while the others do not.

The scale of mortuary feasts among the lower-middle castes is next only to that among the upper-middle castes. The host among the lower-middle castes invites at least one member from each household belonging to castes other than his own. As the food is *pacca*, the problem of pollution is ruled out. All members of a household may be invited if the host has close ties with it. Every member of the host's caste residing in the village is, of course, invited. In this way the total number of invitees from the village are less than those invited by the upper-middle castes. Among the lower castes the scale of feasting is even lower as the higher castes do not accept their food. Their feast thus involves only the lower castes residing in the village in case of *gānv ghātḍi* and those in the *chautāḷo* in case of *nyāt*.[2] The upper castes have reduced drastically the scale of feasting on account of 'social reforms' adopted by them in recent times. The mortuary feast is organized only for about 20 persons besides family members. A few Saads, Saamis and Brahmins, i.e., members of the priestly castes, are invited to the feast for religious merit.

### *Recent Changes in Caste Hierarchy*

Caste ranking has been affected by many changes in the relation between caste and occupation in the post-independence period. Recent developments in the industrial and other sectors have opened new and alternative economic opportunities to some people. The traditional callings and current occupations of various castes in Mogra are listed in Table 1.4. These are true of a majority of members but not necessarily of every one of them.

The abolition of the feudal land tenure system of *jagirdari* in 1952 has adversely affected the dominance of the upper castes, especially Charans and Rajputs. The other three categories no longer depend on upper caste patronages. They own and cultivate land besides carrying on with their traditional arts, crafts, wage work or other services. This change seems to have taken place almost all over Rajasthan, as can be seen from Chakravarti's (1975) study, which provides detailed description of the decline in authority of the erstwhile *jagirdar* castes, and the emerging new patterns of authority, in village study in north-eastern Rajasthan

[2] The hierarchy within each category of castes has not been explained.

TABLE 1.4 *Traditional calling and main and subsidiary occupations by caste*

| *Caste* | *Traditional calling* | *Current main occupation* | *Subsidiary occupation* |
|---|---|---|---|
| Bania | Trader | Trading | Moneylending |
| Bhambi | Leather worker | Wage labour | Agriculture, other manual work, government service |
| Bhangi | Scavenger | Scavenging | Agriculture, wage labour |
| Bhil | Guard | Government service | Wage labour, poultry keeping |
| Brahmin | Priest | Agriculture | Priestly duties, animal husbandry wage labour |
| Charan | Bard/landlord | Government service | Land leasing, animal husbandry |
| Darjee | Tailor | Tailoring | Agriculture, animal husbandry |
| Daroga | Servant of Rajput | Government service | Agriculture |
| Dholi | Drummer | Drumming | Agriculture, wage labour |
| Jat | Cultivator | Agriculture | Animal husbandry, wage labour, urban service |
| Kareegar (Suthar) | Carpenter | Agriculture/ carpentry | Animal husbandry, petty business |
| Kumbar | Potter | Agriculture | Petty trading, animal husbandry |
| Lawar | Blacksmith | Wage labour | Blacksmithy, agriculture |
| Nai | Barber | Hair cutting | Agriculture, cooking for feasts, attending at weddings |
| Patel | Cultivator | Agriculture | Animal husbandry, petty trading, wage labour, government service |
| Raika | Shepherd | Sheep tending | Agriculture, wage labour |
| Rajput | Ruler/warrior | Agriculture | Animal husbandry, business |
| Saad | Mendicant–Vaishnavite | Agriculture | Priestly duties, wage labour, petty trading, animal husbandry |
| Saami | Mendicant–Shaivite | Agriculture | Priestly duties, wage labour, petty trading, animal husbandry |
| Sargara | Menial servant | Wage labour | Agriculture, wage labour, other manual work |
| Sonar | Goldsmith | Goldsmithy | Agriculture, wage labour |
| Teli (Muslim) | Oil presser | Oil pressing | Tailoring, embroidery, agriculture |
| Vishnoi | Cultivator | Agriculture | Wage labour, driving |

(cf. also Sharma 1974). However, although the Charans and Rajputs in Mogra have lost their old feudal rights and privileges, they continue to hold large tracts of land which they lease out to others. They also continue to maintain a certain traditional life-style. Very few of them, for example, cultivate land themselves.

Charans and Rajputs continue to be dominant also due to their access to formal education and consequent *naukri* (urban salaried jobs). A few of them hold such jobs as peons, bus conductors, policemen, teachers and office clerks. One of them is a college lecturer. They continue to have substantial interest in land. Most of them, in fact, commute between the village and their work-place. So they derive income from land rent and urban salaries. Most of their women raise cattle and/or goats to supplement income by selling milk.

Patel and Jat are the traditional peasant castes. They were tillers of land and their main calling is agriculture on their own land. While the abolition of feudal land tenures has led to downward mobility of Charans and Rajputs, it has helped upward mobility of Patels and Jats. With 163 out of 410 (40%) households, the Patels compete with Charans for dominance.

As shown in Table 1.4, most members of the artisan and service castes (constituting the lower-middle category) continue to engage in their traditional calling, while others engage in wage labour, petty trading and agriculture. With the abolition of *jagirs* and the consequent displacement of *jajmani* relations, the artisan castes took to agriculture on a larger scale than in the past (cf. Pocock 1962, and Mahobia 1976). In his study of the semi-arid region in Rajasthan (in which Mogra lies), Jodha (1985) highlights how abolition of *jagirs* affected the artisans and their traditional crafts. Consequently, they have taken to agriculture as well for additional income.

A similar shift is found among the lower castes. The Bhambis in Mogra and the neighbouring villages have, as a group, ceased to perform the traditional leather work and skinning of dead cattle in an attempt to Sanskritize. All the lower castes engage in agriculture as owner-cultivators, labourers, and sharecroppers, and do non-agricultural wage work, primarily as construction workers.

The phenomenon of village people frequently engaging in occupations other than those traditionally ascribed to their caste, is complex and has to be seen both at the individual and the household levels. One or more members from several households in different castes have ventured into various new occupations owing to urbanization and modernization. Some have taken up trading in goods and commodities as their principal occupation, while the rest of the household does agriculture, animal husbandry, etc. Many young boys are skilled and unskilled workers in factories in urban centres. Several others hold jobs in public and private sector establishments as teachers, clerks, accountants, factory hands, shop assistants, etc. Almost all persons in white collar jobs belong to the younger generation while their parents and other senior family members continue with their traditional calling. Of the 79 urban job holders, only two were old enough to have formally retired (at the age of 58 years), while the rest continue to work.

The Charans hold the majority of white collar government jobs, while the other castes are found more in private sector services. Salaried jobs taken up by educated people are considered more prestigious than traditional callings in Mogra. In addition to Charans, members of other castes have also taken up salaried and non-traditional jobs, which has further complicated the hierarchical order of castes in Mogra.

Numerical strength is important in a political system with adult franchise. The Patels have gained political importance owing to their numerical strength too. They constitute nearly one-half of the village population. In local level politics, especially representation in the village panchayat, Patels have taken the lead. A Patel has been elected as *sarpanch* (head of the statutory panchayat). In addition, the numerical preponderance of Patels as well as other upper-middle castes in the village has made them near equal to the erstwhile dominant Charan and Rajput castes.

### *The Village Economy*

Agriculture continues to be the mainstay. All castes have taken up some agricultural work or other besides their traditional occupations as shown in Table 1.4. Every household in the village, except that of a Bania trader, is involved in agriculture, as owner-cultivator, tenant, sharecropper or labourer. Most households own land, although there are large variations in the extent of ownership. Those with no or little land have leased it for cultivation.

The holdings range from 2.5 to 106 acres, the average being 20–25 acres. Patel, Jat and Charan are the major land-owning castes, although artisan and scheduled castes also own some land. There are 64 households without land. Most of them are Raika (shepherd) or untouchable. A few landless households are found even among the Patel, Brahmin, Saad Darjee, and other castes. Except for Charans and Rajputs, all others cultivate land as tenants and sharecroppers, especially if their own holding is small.

Much of the cultivation is carried out with household labour.[3] During the peak agricultural season there exists a system of labour exchange (*dīlāvaḍi*) between households to meet labour requirement. Wage labour is used only as a last resort. A few large farmers employ farm servants (*haḷi*) on an annual contract basis. Employing a *haḷi* is not viable for small farmers. People prefer hiring wage labour occasionally to employing a *haḷi*. A few cultivators employ tractor drivers on a contractual basis during the agricultural season usually for three or four months from May-June onwards. This is the case especially with large farmers who do not have grown up son(s) to help them manage the tractors. The upper castes rarely work as *haḷis* or tractor drivers. However, Brahmins do take up wage labour in agriculture, unlike Banias, Charans and Rajputs. Most of the wage labourers are from landless households of the untouchable, artisan and shepherd castes. Wage labour is hired only during utmost need, because it involves cash payment and often an advance payment to ensure attendance. By avoiding *haḷi* and wage labour, a household saves on cash expenditure.[4] This society values earning and saving rather than spending money on hired labour.

---

[3] Prabhakara and Usha (1986) show on the basis of National Sample Survey data a very high proportion of unpaid helpers in rural Rajasthan: 34.4% of the total rural population as compared to the all India figure of 13.5%. Regular farm servants and bonded labourers are also less common in Rajasthan: 0.91% as compared to the all India average of 2.97% of the total rural population.

[4] This may be explained by two factors: first, low rainfall and low productivity do not make bonded labour on farms an economic proposition. Also, the wage rate is very high. A farm servant may cost about Rs 2,000 annually in addition to

Almost all agriculture in Mogra is dry and dependent on the monsoon. Rainfall is scanty and uncertain. The peasant reaps on an average one good crop in three years. A good crop is one that can keep the household going for more than a year. Whatever grass grows during the poorer monsoon years is collected for fodder. Land here is less fertile than in southern and eastern Rajasthan. *Bajra* is the staple cereal. Lentils, cluster-beans and sesame are other crops. Since agriculture is dependent on rainfall, only one major crop can be grown on most of the land. Irrigation is scarce. Land is irrigated only with well water and it is possible to raise an additional crop. The households owning irrigated land have ventured into the cultivation of wheat, black mustard and vegetables.

The bulk of agricultural produce is for consumption at home and for the cattle. Some is sold to buy tea, sugar, salt, clothing, utensils, jewellery, building material, tools, etc. Agriculture is not prosperous enough to support advanced technology, although recently some people have acquired modern agricultural machines. There are 39 tractors, two fodder-cutting machines, and two pumps to lift water from wells for irrigation. The use of hybrid seeds is gaining popularity. Organic manure is largely used. Chemical fertilizers are sparingly applied.

Animal husbandry is the most common allied or subsidiary activity. A few decades ago milk selling was considered a lowly venture. It was like selling one's son. Now most households keep cows and buffaloes with the explicit purpose of selling milk.

The members of a household practise more than one subsidiary occupation simultaneously. For instance, a Patel household runs a tea shop, a flour mill and a fair-price shop besides doing agriculture and animal husbandry. Although the Bania trader lends money on a large scale, moneylending can be practised by anyone with spare money irrespective of caste. I found a Patel and a Bhambi lending money, albeit on a smaller scale than the Bania.

For the last decade and a half, non-agricultural wage labour,

---

food, clothing, maintenance and small payments in kind to the servant's family now and then. Secondly, women and even children work on farms along with men.

especially for construction is in demand in Jodhpur city and the area around Mogra. The contractors offer free transportation. A large proportion of untouchables is engaged in such work. Their dependence on the higher castes in the village is, therefore, decreasing. They prefer agricultural work only when they get proper wages. Members of higher castes have to call on them at their homes and often pay some advance amount. The nature of traditional interdependence between the lower and the other castes in Mogra is thus gradually changing.

### *The Household Economy*

Men, women and children have different roles in the household economy characterized by multiple callings. The division of labour is based usually on age, sex and social position. Economically the most active age group is 16–45 years. However, people do not retire at 45. Physical fitness is an important criterion in deciding whether a person can work or not after this age. During peak agricultural seasons, it is only physical inability that decides absence from work on fields. By the time parents reach their fifties, their grown up and married sons, their wives and children take over the major share of work in the house and on the fields. The old parents do less strenuous work.

Men do almost all the tasks associated with agriculture and wage labour. They plough, sow, weed, harvest, thrash, winnow and transport produce home. They take grain, fodder and fuel-wood to the city for sale. They buy most of the household provisions, seeds, tools, etc. They cut branches for making tools and household furniture. They manure the fields and keep a watch on them, especially at nights and the early mornings. They clear the fields of larger bushes. They dig trenches around fields and make fences. Maintenance and construction of houses is done both by men and women, though men never plaster the houses with dung paste. Older men usually baby sit their grandchildren but rarely their own children as it is considered immodest.

Men do various jobs associated with cattle raising. They clear the feeding troughs. They make and repair barns. They cut fodder by hand and/or arrange the fodder-cutting machines. They make almost all the arrangements for hiring tractors for various jobs on and off the fields. Filling of underground water storages (*tanko*) in the house with the help of tractors is also their job. Shepherds take their herds to the neighbouring districts and even beyond during the non-agricultural period. One or two women join a group of around 10 men and move out together.

Men in salaried jobs are occupied most of the day. Many of them commute to their places of work on bicycle. During holidays, they take over most tasks generally performed by other men in the house, the cattle shed and the fields. During the peak agricultural season, they take leave from their offices to help the households when more labour is required. In addition, they spend a great deal of time in meeting others in the village, gossiping at tea stalls, shops, etc.

Among all castes, work in the household and the cattle shed is largely a woman's responsibility. This is in addition to the bearing and rearing of children, managing the house, and working out all details to keep the kitchen going. They milk and feed cattle, clean the shed, make dung cakes, smear the house with dung and mud paste at regular intervals, cook, wash utensils and clothes, and clean the house and the street in front. They do all kinds of food processing, such as chaffing, pounding, grinding, and fetching water and fuel. They process and store certain food items for the whole year. The young daughters-in-law take up strenuous chores, while the mothers-in-law do the lighter ones. In addition, women work on farms and engage in wage labour. The extent and nature of their role in agriculture is linked to the customary practice of *purdo* (*purdah*, literally, curtain) i.e., seclusion. Women of the Charan and Rajput castes do not work in the fields for this reason, while those of other castes do.

The Charan and Rajput women observe *purdo*. They usually remain indoors. Whenever they move out, they wrap a sheet around them. Another manifestation of female seclusion is *gūngto*, a veil to cover the face, worn by women of all castes. A young daughter-in-law covers her face in the presence of all seniors (male and female) in the conjugal household, the neighbourhood and even the village, unless the elderly man is a natal kin. A daughter-in-law does not speak directly even with elderly women until several years after marriage. She nods her head or clicks her tongue to convey short responses (usually 'yes' and 'no' respectively), especially when no child is around to assist her in communicating with senior conjugal relatives. She may do so only after bearing two to three children while still observing *gūngto*. It is only after becoming a mother-in-law and a grandmother that she can remove her *gūngto*, and that too before senior women.

Except for Charan and Rajput women, all other women join their men in agricultural and non-agricultural work. Peasant and artisan women usually work on their family farms or on leased lands. They generally avoid doing wage labour elsewhere, unless forced by famine or some calamity. Except for ploughing and sowing, women do chores like weeding, harvesting and clearing the fields. They help men in fencing, and all other tasks involved in reaping the crop and taking it home. Although women work alongside men in most of the strenuous tasks, they abstain from certain cognate tasks like ploughing. Similarly, Kumbar women do not make pots and pans, though they procure mud and process it. With the introduction of tractors, ploughing, sowing and transporting have become, by and large, male jobs. Women mostly carry loads on head.

Childbearing and rearing are not seen as hindrances to chores at home and on the field. It is not uncommon for a woman to resume work a week after child delivery. She is a beast of burden working on land throughout the day. She wakes up before all others early in the morning to work at home and in the cattle-shed and to take care of children before leaving for the fields. After returning from a days's work alongside men, she resumes her work —tending the home, cattle and children before going to bed.

Women do a considerable amount of grain processing after the produce is brought home. Grain is graded into categories for seed, domestic use and for sale if there is an excess. Semi-formed grains which are mixed with nodes are sorted out by women for human and animal consumption. This is to be done for each type of crop—bajra, jowar and lentils, because people grow two to four crops simultaneously on their fields rather than specialize in just one. This work is done even by Charan and Rajput women, as it does not demand stepping out of the house.

Women among the upper-middle, lower-middle and lower

castes perform back-breaking tasks for their households. In order to get social and emotional acceptance in the conjugal family, the woman works hard in as well as outside the house. However, motherhood is the final cementing factor, especially the birth of a son. The lower caste women also work hard. They do all the household duties besides wage labour. They do domestic chores fast to be available for wage labour in time. Restrictions of time are imposed on labourers by others. For peasant women the time is set by senior household members.

In addition to working on land as sharecroppers and labourers, lower caste women work as construction labourers. For the last several years a few contractors have made arrangements to pick up labourers from Mogra in the morning to construction sites and bring them back in the evening. Women hurry up their household chores to be ready for work by 8 a. m. They return around seven in the evening. This routine is followed almost throughout the year with some gaps during the monsoons, when the demand for labour on land increases. Wages for work on land are more than for non-agricultural work. During the harvesting season of 1984, wages shot up to Rs 20 and 25 against the non-agricultural wage of Rs 10 and 12 per day for women and men respectively.

Children also contribute to the household economy. It is more indirect between 5–10 years of age. They take on small tasks like baby sitting, keeping a watch on birds, cats and dogs, fetching a glass of water and running errands. Their help relieve the elders for more productive activities. After the age of 10, children gradually begin to help elders more directly. They assist the seniors in various chores in and outside the house.

The tasks performed by small children in the village and the town cannot be equated. While the latter are rightly called labourers, most of the jobs done by village children are a mixture of play and work. For instance, children, especially small girls, look after their younger siblings and cousins. But they rarely baby sit in isolation within closed doors. They leave the young ones on the streets at one place and play among themselves. They suspend the game as and when the younger ones need attention. If a child is not attended to by the older sibling, the others in the play group point it out. If an adult passes by, he/she yells at the older sibling to come and attend to the child. The mother is thus left free to do other chores.

Children around the age of 10 tend cattle. They take them out to graze. Groups of children jointly do this task. Children also take cattle for watering to the village pond. They occasionally serve fodder to the younger cattle. They collect dung, twigs and firewood for the household. Groups of children, especially girls, go to the village *hīm* or to the nearby fields and return with head-loads of twigs almost daily throughout the summer. Fuel has to be stored for the rainy season, as jobs on land hardly leave any time for collecting fuel, nor does wet fuel burn easily. Small girls are commonly seen collecting dung from wherever possible. They devote a great deal of time looking out for, and collecting, scarcely available fuel. children are often encouraged to sneak into others' fields for dried cowdung, twigs and branches. A few parents send their girls with a bowl on their heads to collect dung while they take cattle for watering to the village pond.

Children, especially girls, are helpful in fetching water from the pond or the well when the pond dries during summer. On an average two to three pitchers are brought twice a day in each household of 4–5 members. Initial training is with iron or brass pots. Later, they graduate to earthern pitchers. It is an important part of every girl's training to learn to fetch water. Mothers are rarely lax in this respect. It also saves on the expenditure of filling the *tānko* at quick intervals. Rarely do boys and men fetch water in pitchers on their shoulders. They place them on bullock carts instead. But raising bullocks has become too expensive, and very few own them. Nowadays some people get a *tānko* built in their house or cattle shed, and water containers are brought on tractors, own or hired. This reduces a woman's water fetching burden though she still makes one or two rounds of water-fetching on her heads even if there is a *tānko* at home.

Girls of 10–12 years usually cook the evening meal, epecially during peak agricultural seasons. By this age, they also learn to milk, feed and tether the cows. They perform light tasks in the fields, like weeding and carrying younger siblings to and from the fields, while their mothers carry grass loads for the cattle.

Scaring birds away from fields and keeping a vigil (*rukāḷo*; literally, protection on the fields) is a time-consuming task.

Younger children walk through fields using slings for this purpose. Usually a household has fields scattered around the village rather than at one place. As many persons are required for *rukāḷo* as the number of fields cultivated. Children are mostly assigned *rukāḷo* as it is uneconomical to get such jobs done by hired hands or by household elders. It is not easy to hire labour for *rukāḷo* at odd hours. The peak hours of *rukāḷo* are early morning and evening when birds raid fields.

Boys take up most of the male tasks by the time they are 15–16 years old. Their training begins at an early age. School-going boys have to assist in househld tasks before and after school hours. A typical case of a peasant boy who combines education with household and other work is described below.

> Dalia, an 11-year-old Patel boy, is a student in the fifth class. He lays out fodder for cattle in troughs and takes his cattle to the village pond for a drink twice a day. His younger brother, Bhalia, aged nine, goes with him as the herd is rather large. Dalia herds in the cattle in the evening on their return. His 13-year-old sister helps him tether the cattle in the shed (*vāḍa*). During the cropping season his sister, who does not go to school, takes the cattle for grazing. She saves on expenses for a *haḷi*. Dalia often helps her to fetch water. His younger brother Kalia takes the goats for grazing. Dalia has learnt to drive the household tractor and wants to be in command. He drove the tractor for three nights while they were spreading manure on the fields. 'If I drive the tractor, my father can help my uncles in loading and spreading manure. Even one man's contribution makes a difference. I sleep the whole morning and afternoon to drive at night'. Since his father is illiterate, he helps his father keep the tractor accounts in a small note book. He writes whatever his father instructs him to. He also goes to the fields with his mother and sister to clear the fields for ploughing and making a fence around them. 'I want to do all these tasks before the school reopens. Once I start going to school, I will not be able to spare enough time for the fields. My mother and grandparents persuade me to stay back but I don't want to miss school'.

Dalia's case highlights children's contribution to the household economy. They are encouraged to emulate their elders and work hard in the larger interest of the household. They receive parental and neighbourhood appreciation for hard work. Children's hard work enhances the status of the household. This is similar to the economic relevance of children in a Javanese village

(White 1975). He argues that a large number of people does not mean they are mostly reduced to complete idleness. On the contrary, each is forced to work harder and for increasingly long hours.

By the age of 12, girls learn to clean the grain of stones, and chaff and grind (or semi-grind) them, in a hand mill. They learn to clean the cattle shed and the house and make dung cakes. They are also encouraged to learn some craft like embroidery, bead work, cloth repair, making beds from rags and pitcher stands to fetch water. All these are done usually during the non-agricultural season. Girls assist in house repair, smearing the floors and walls with dung paste, colouring the walls, and making designs on them. Wool spinning is done mostly by Raika girls and women. Artisan children learn traditional crafts like tailoring, carpentry smithy and pottery from their parents and other elders.

> Mangloji, an old potter recalls that he has done pottery all his life for survival, i.e., he took charge too early in life. 'My father died when I was 11. Being the eldest child, I had to take up the whole responsibility. Gradually I could manage all the affairs of this craft.'

Children aged 6–7 years are a great asset to parents. They lend a helping hand in numerous domestic chores, such as work in the cattle shed and on the fields, and assistance in looking after younger siblings. When a daughter is about 10, she is made to learn almost all the tasks that women perform. By the time of *muklāwo* she is fully trained to take up women's chores in and outside the house. The value of a daughter is expressed in the proverb, *Bēti ri maa rāṇi ne būdāpē bhare paṇi* (literally, a daughter's mother is a queen but has to fetch water in old age). The proverb also suggests, subtely, the need for a son whose wife would take over household tasks when the daughter leaves her natal home upon *muklawo*.

People appreciate hard working tender children. If children do not learn expected jobs, they and their parents are criticized. Some people, especially near relatives, criticize them to their face, while others do so behind their back.

> Keli, a Patel woman and her 10-year-old daughter, Saao, are frequently cited as examples by many women in the neighbourhood for not behaving the way they should. A neighbour said, 'Keli is a

> strange mother. She is spoiling her daughter. She has no skills to teach her daughter to help her, and she does not even make dung cakes. We never see her cooking or milking. Her daughter will always be scolded in her conjugal household. Keli will be remembered as a mother who was careless about her daughter's training.' Once Keli explained to a few women who were critical of her daughter while they sat in her courtyard: 'She has been saving Rs 700 a year for the past two years. I did not have to pay a *haḷi* for grazing cattle. She cooks sometimes. I don't allow her to make dung cakes because she spoils them and I cannot afford to waste dung like that'. But the other women were not convinced. One of them said: 'She may spoil the dung here but she cannot afford to do it at her inlaws' house.'

The household elders, relatives and neighbours teach children to help parents. Adults in the community engage themselves frequently in evaluation and comparision of the children's performance. This helps in making children emulate adults in work in and outside the house.

Children make an important contribution to the household economy through their hard work, and help enhance its economic and social status. As labour is highly valued and there is little mechanization, parents and children work together for the household.

CHAPTER 2

# *A Profile of Ever Married Women and their Fertility*

Most of the data pertaining to fertility experiences here is collected from ever married women in Mogra. The term 'ever married woman' means one who has been married at least once, but is not necessarily married presently (i.e., at the time of fieldwork). Thus, ever married women in Mogra include all married, widowed, divorced and separated women. These also include 17 remarried women, whose duration of first marriage and children then born form part of their total marital and fertility experience.

Since women are bearers of children and share the major responsibility of rearing them, it is necessary to elicit information directly from them rather than on their behalf from other persons. Hence the emphasis on women respondents who had first-hand experience of reproduction. Also, the initial stages of fieldwork revealed that husbands are discouraged from showing any overt interest in their wives' and children's affairs pertaining to illness, clothing, social visits and so on for several years after marriage. Of necessity, therefore, women are at the centre of this inquiry which is not restricted only to the respondents' experiences during the period of fieldwork, but is extended into their past experiences too. As women undergo the experience of bearing children, they are better able to recall their fertility experiences.

The data on ever married women is obtained from household census, interviews with the women, and from participant observation. In all there are 693 women respondents. I have also interviewed 20 widowers about the reproductive experiences of their deceased wives. I cross-checked this data with their close relatives. Although 20 cases are a very small number, the data on them makes for more complete coverage. Thus, while there are 693 respondents, one may say there are 20 subjects, making a total of 713 cases of ever married women. Computations, such as the number of children born, dead and surviving, are worked out with reference to all the 713 women.

My being a woman researcher helped immensely in the study. It enabled me easy and greater access to the world of women rather than that of men. I could not collect much information from men. This should not mean that I have information only about women. As marriage and childbearing and rearing involve both men and women, I have not ignored men totally. On numerous occasions, while I interviewed women, their husbands were present and keen to provide information. Several others, including friends, neighbours and children, were also present. They reinforced, contradicted or added information in response to my questions. Participant observation gave an insight into men's behaviour.

Here, numerical data along critical demographic and social variables concerning 713 ever married women is presented and discussed. This relates to marriage, motherhood, number of children born, dead and surviving, mother-in-lawhood, caste, household type, economic status, education, etc. I am aware that the data could have been treated with greater statistical sophistication. I am unable to do so. Also, my primary aim remains a thick description of the logistics of fertility behaviour. The simplistic presentation of numerical data purports to portray a bare picture of the field as it exists. The idea is to provide a general background about fertility behaviour which is discussed more deeply and intensively in later chapters.

Table 2.1 shows the marital status of the 713 women. Marriage is near universal in Mogra. Over 82% of the women are currently married (including 17 remarried women), and 14.72% are widows. There is only one divorced woman. (Her former husband died after she was divorced. She is not categorized as a 'widow' here to retain this feature of social reality.) There is one deserted woman. She was turned out by her husband upon his marriage with another

TABLE 2.1 *Distribution of women by marital status*

| *Marital status* | *Women* | |
|---|---|---|
| | *Number* | *%* |
| Married | 586 | 82.19 |
| Widowed | 105 | 14.72 |
| Divorced | 1 | 0.14 |
| Deserted | 1 | 0.14 |
| Dead | 20 | 2.81 |
| Total | 713 | 100.00 |

woman. The table shows 20 dead women. The reason for their inclusion in the sample and the source of data on them have already been discussed.

The percentage of widowed, divorced and separated women in Mogra (15%) is higher than that (8.6%) for rural India as a whole. The percentage of widowed, divorced and separated men in Mogra, namely, 2.81, is however very close to that (2.97) for rural India (see Census of India, 1981b, Part II Special, Statement 7: 34).

Age at widow/widowerhood is an important dimension of fertility behaviour. Table 2.2 provides this data in respect of 105 widows, one divorced and one separated woman, and 20

TABLE 2.2 *Widows and widowers by age at widow/widowerhood*

| *Age at widow/widowerhood (in years)* | *Widows* | *Widowers* |
|---|---|---|
| Up to 20 | 3 | 0 |
| 21–25 | 7 | 1 |
| 26–30 | 13 | 1 |
| 31–35 | 14 | 3 |
| 36–40 | 8 | 3 |
| 41–45 | 11 | 3 |
| 46–50 | 12 | 0 |
| 51–55 | 14 | 2 |
| 56–60 | 15 | 3 |
| 61+ | 10 | 4 |
| Total | 107 | 20 |

widowers. Only 10 widows lost their husbands at an early age, i.e., before they crossed the age of 25. In all, 50% of women lost their husbands before crossing the age of 40, and the rest later. The number of widowers (20) is quite small. This is mainly due to the higher incidence of remarriage among widowers than among widows. Besides, longer survival of women after crossing the reproductive age is a well known fact in demography. In Mogra, only one man lost his wife before crossing the age of 25, and 40% of all widowers lost theirs' before they were 40.

Table 2.3 shows the distribution of 713 women and their husbands by age. Information on the ages of 20 deceased women and 107 deceased men was obtained from their spouses and relatives. Their ages are recorded as what they were at the time of death. Thus, the ages of as many as 127 persons included in Table 2.3 were not recorded simultaneously with those of the currently married 586 persons, i.e., at the end of 1984, the time of my field census. Also, the time between their death and the year 1984 has little relevance for fertility analysis.

TABLE 2.3 *Distribution of women and their husbands by age*

| *Age (in years)* | *Women* | | *Women's husbands* | |
|---|---|---|---|---|
| | *Number* | % | *Number* | % |
| Below 15 | 6 | 0.84 | 1 | 0.14 |
| 16–20 | 85 | 11.92 | 42 | 5.89 |
| 21–25 | 107 | 15.01 | 89 | 12.48 |
| 26–30 | 130 | 18.23 | 119 | 16.69 |
| 31–35 | 68 | 9.54 | 83 | 11.64 |
| 36–40 | 77 | 10.80 | 86 | 12.06 |
| 41–45 | 51 | 7.15 | 70 | 9.82 |
| 46–50 | 48 | 6.73 | 56 | 7.85 |
| 51–55 | 30 | 4.21 | 47 | 6.60 |
| 56–60 | 53 | 7.43 | 53 | 7.44 |
| 61+ | 58 | 8.13 | 67 | 9.40 |
| Total | 713 | 100.00 | 713 | 100.00 |

Almost 80% of the women are aged between 15 and 50, i.e., the reproductive age group. Those above 50 (who have crossed their reproductive age) are less in number. Similarly, over 70% of the husbands are aged between 15 and 55. An in-built bias of such age distribution is that fewer older people are available, due to low life expectency, to give information about their past fertility, say 50 years ago.

I have classified castes in Mogra into four categories in the preceding chapter. Table 2.4 shows the distribution of 713 women by these four categories. Women belonging to upper-middle castes, Jat, Patel, Raika and Vishnoi, are the largest in number (60.87%), followed by those of lower-middle and lower castes, each constituting roughly 15% of the total. The upper caste women are the smallest in number, 9.12%.

TABLE 2.4 *Distribution of women by caste categories*

| *Caste category* | *Women* | |
|---|---|---|
| | *Number* | % |
| Upper | 65 | 9.12 |
| Upper-middle | 434 | 60.87 |
| Lower-middle | 109 | 15.29 |
| Lower | 105 | 14.73 |
| Total | 713 | 100.00 |

As mentioned in Chapter 1, people follow their traditional callings besides engaging in one or more other occupations. Certain jobs are done customarily by men and others by women. Different members of the same household are often engaged in different tasks. Table 2.5 shows the distribution of 713 ever married women by their principal calling or by the economic activity they did for most of their active life. In addition, it shows the principal calling of their husbands. Wage labour includes construction and agricultural work done for wages; skilled work includes that of artisans; agriculture means cultivation other than for wages; animal husbandry refers to the raising of cows, buffaloes, sheep, goats and camels; business means trading of all kinds; salaried jobs include those in private and public organizations of a

TABLE 2.5 *Distribution of 713 women and their husbands by their principal calling/occupation*

| *Principal calling* | *Women* | | *Women's husbands* | |
|---|---|---|---|---|
| | *Number* | % | *Number* | % |
| Unskilled wage work | 46 | 6.5 | 38 | 5.3 |
| Skilled work | 22 | 3.1 | 73 | 10.2 |
| Agriculture | 542 | 76.0 | 445 | 62.4 |
| Animal husbandry | 53 | 7.4 | 58 | 8.1 |
| Business | — | — | 20 | 2.8 |
| Salaried job | 02 | 0.3 | 79 | 11.1 |
| Household work | 48 | 6.7 | — | — |
| Total | 713 | 100.0 | 713 | 100.0 |

non-agricultural kind; and household work consists of unpaid work done at home.

Table 2.5 shows the occupations of 713 women and their husbands but not those of their households, although in some, more than one person may be engaged in the same occupation. In all the occupational categories, the callings of women and their husbands do not always coincide. The number of women in unskilled labour is slightly higher (46 women against 38 men), while only 22 women compared to 73 men are engaged in skilled labour. More women (542) than men (445) are engaged in agriculture. On the other hand, slightly more men (58) than women (53) are occupied in animal husbandry. No woman is engaged in business in contrast to 20 men. Conversely, no man has household work as his occupation against 48 women. Men (79) dominate in salaried jobs compared to women (2). These two, a nurse and a teacher, are outsiders living in Mogra.

### *Household and Family*

People in Mogra follow the patrivirilocal rule at marriage. That is, the son brings his wife upon marriage to reside with his parents. Traditionally, every Hindu couple aspires to preside over a household with several married sons, their wives and children. This gives them enormous satisfaction and status in society. Separation of households and partition of property between married brothers is expected to take place ideally after the death of both parents. But the ideal is not always met in practice. Married sons do secede to form their own nuclear households even during their parents' lifetime.

It is important to distinguish between family and household. While a household is a residential and commensal unit, a family is not necessarily so. A family may be composed of more than one household. For example, when the parents and their married son live in two separate households, they continue to constitute a family. Similarly, with two brothers living in separate households.

Households belong to different types depending on their demographic and kinship composition and the phases of the developmental process. On the basis of their kinship composition they are of two major types, simple and complex (Shah 1973). The distinction between them appears to be similar, but not identical, to that between nuclear and joint families. A simple household with a married couple and their unmarried children is considered a nuclear family. But the addition of other relatives, such as a daughter-in-law and son's children makes it a joint family. So the household becomes complex. However, deletion of any one or more members from a simple household would still keep it simple. For instance, a household of one man or woman is categorized as simple. Similarly, households consisting of only a married couple, or only of siblings, or of mother with unmarried children are all sub-types of a simple household, although they do not form complete nuclear families. The addition to a simple household of a member belonging to another simple household (for example, a married daughter, son's wife's sibling, etc.) makes it a complex one. For instance, parents with a married son, his wife and unmarried children, or parents with unmarried children and father's siblings, are some of the sub-types of complex households.

Of the 410 households in Mogra, 215 (52.43%) are simple and 195 (47.57%) complex. Table 2.6 shows that although 52.43% households are simple, only 30.15% of the 713 ever married women reside in them. The remaining 69.85% married women live in complex households, constituting 47.57% of all households.

TABLE 2.6 *Distribution of ever married women by household type*

| *Household type* | *Households* | | *Ever married women* | |
|---|---|---|---|---|
| | *Number* | *%* | *Number* | *%* |
| Simple | 215 | 52.43 | 215 | 30.15 |
| Complex | 195 | 47.57 | 498 | 69.85 |
| Total | 410 | 100.00 | 713 | 100.00 |

In other words, of the 713 ever married women, 215 women and their husbands live in simple households, i.e., one couple per household. On the other hand, 498 married women live in 195 complex households, i.e., roughly 2.5 couples per household. Thus, for every one ever married woman living along with her husband and unmarried children in a simple household, at least two women live along with their husband and/or children in a complex household. In some complex households there may be more than two couples.

The average size of a simple household is five members and that of a complex household 8.5, while the average size of the two together is 6.7, which is the same as that for 192 villages in Jodhpur *tehsil* in 1981 (District Census Handbook—Jodhpur 1981c). This is larger than the average of 5.9 for rural Rajasthan and 5.5 for rural India in 1981 (based on household population by religion of head of household, Census of India 1981d, Series 1, Paper 4 of 1984. See also Kolenda's 1989 exhaustive account of joint family households in rural Rajasthan).

The developmental process of the household as delineated by Shah (1973) is a major contribution to the field of family studies. It overcomes the common misunderstanding that the Indian family is either nuclear or joint. The concept of the developmental process looks at the household as a dynamic and not a static unit. Shah observes that a household constantly undergoes the processes of progression and regression. He states:

> The progressive development of a household takes place with an increase in membership, mainly by birth, in-marriage of women, and return of out-married women and their husbands or children.

> The regressive development takes place with a decrease in membership, by death, out-marriage of women, return of in-married women and their husbands or children, and partition (1973: 82).

Separation of households in Mogra may take place during the lifetime of parents when married sons (i.e., brothers) and their wives cannot get along with each other. But at least one son will remain with his parents. Separation of a lone son from his parents is almost impossible. The only exception is a Patel who lives separately from his old widowed mother. He has divorced his wife, and delinked himself from his mother. Only 303 of the 713 ever married women considered here, have separated from complex households to form their own simple ones. There are many households where more than one married son live jointly with their old parents. In a few households as many as five married sons do so which raises the prestige of the household enormously.

It is rare for a newly-married couple to establish a new household (see Kolenda 1989 for joint family households in Rajasthan) because the adolescent husband is largely dependent on his parents and other household elders for his subsistence which comes from working on the household land, cattle, etc., Even if the boy has an independent source of income, he remits most of it to his parents, and is dependent on them for various other things. His social and emotional dependence on the parents persists for quite a few years. Also, if he resides in a city for a job, he usually keeps his wife and/ or children with his parents in the village. It is only a few years after marriage—by which time he has a few children—that he attains some authority to establish a separate household. While the time range for separation is up to 51 years, the highest number (26) have occurred during the tenth year of marriage. Of the 303 separations, 154 have taken place between 4 and 12 years of marriage. The majority of those separating within three years belong to the lower castes.

Separate arrangement for cooking is the minimum prerequisite for a household's separation to be effective. Usually a separate room or sometimes even a corner in the house is used as a kitchen by the couple keen on separation. Eventually a part of the house is demarcated for the seceding couple and their children, unless the house is so congested that division is not possible. In which case, the seceding couple shift to another site belonging to the household and construct a house and a cattle shed. Hence, most brothers and near agnates live adjacent to each other, usually on the same street, as mentioned in Chapter 1.

As there is a time lag between marriage and household separation, the seceding son's wife bears one or more children while living in the complex household. She may also have one or more children after seceding from it. Thus, a woman's fertility career can span different household types. This point is further elaborated while discussing Tables 2.19 and 2.20.

The marriage of sons and the arrival of daughters-in-law turns the once simple household into a complex one. Although one houseold separates from another, the family bond between them continues. The process of fission occurs at different stages, and for different reasons, in the developmental process of the household (se Fortes 1958 and Shah 1973 for an elaboration).

The household and the family are vital to its members. Villagers identify themselves with their households in which virtually all their interests are tied up. The community recognizes this identity. A question like, 'Who are you?' is rarely asked. The common question is, 'Whose child are you?' The prime identity is through parents and the household. It is inconceivable for people that an individual's personal character and concerns should not be identified closely with his or her household. Similarly, the exclusive rights of individual ownership of land are rarely recognized and expressed. Properties like house, land, cattle, are said to belong to the household even if they are in the name of the male head of the household in government records. A nuclear family household may be independent economically but not in its social ties with other related households both in and outside the village. That a household may not be functionally independent has been observed by Shah (1973), Ramu (1988) and Kolenda (1989). The household and the family provide to the individual both identity and security. Wiser and Wiser (1963) aptly point out that a man finds wider security within the household and the family to which he belongs despite bitter quarrels.

## *Marriage and Childbirth*

It is customary among all except the upper castes to celebrate marriage by two sets of ceremonies, *vīva* and *muklāwo* (consummation of marriage), the latter following the former usually after a year or more. That only the latter influences fertility needs hardly be pointed out. Most demographic studies on fertility however, assume the wedding ceremony and consummation of marriage as one and the same thing, which then leads to the erroneous conclusion that an early age at marriage leads to high fertility. In this book the terms *muklāwo*, *ano* and marriage are used invariably to connote consummation of marriage. We shall discuss the correlation between age at marriage and fertility in Mogra.

The ages at *vīva* of 713 ever married women are presented in Table 2.7 and their ages as well as those of their husbands' at *muklāwo* in Table 2.8. Over 71% of the girls are wedded before they

TABLE 2.7 *Distribution of women by age at wedding (viva)*

| *Age at wedding (in years)* | *Women* | |
|---|---|---|
| | *Number* | % |
| Up to 5 | 100 | 14.02 |
| 6–10 | 196 | 27.49 |
| 11–15 | 211 | 29.60 |
| 16–20 | 192 | 26.93 |
| 21–25 | 14 | 1.96 |
| Total | 713 | 100.00 |

cross the age of 15, and only 29% after. The average age for marriage (*muklāwo*) of boys and girls is 20.45 and 16.21 years respectively in Mogra, compared with 20.35 and 16.09 years in Rajasthan, and 23.27 and 18.32 years in India in 1981 (Census of India 1981b Part II Special, Statement 11: 37). The age at marriage in Mogra is lower than that prescribed by law, i.e., 18 years for a girl and 21 for a boy.

For how long women remain 'married' and at what age they attain motherhood are closely linked with their age at marriage

TABLE 2.8 *Distribution of women and their husbands by age at marriage (muklawo)*

| *Age at marriage (in years)* | *Women* | | *Men* | |
|---|---|---|---|---|
| | *Number* | % | *Number* | % |
| up to 10 | 2 | 0.28 | 0 | 0 |
| 11–15 | 270 | 37.87 | 55 | 7.71 |
| 16–20 | 422 | 59.19 | 355 | 49.79 |
| 21–25 | 19 | 02.66 | 229 | 32.11 |
| 26–30 | — | — | 53 | 7.44 |
| 31+ | — | — | 21 | 2.95 |
| Total | 713 | 100.00 | 713 | 100.00 |

(see Tables 2.9 and 2.10). Marital duration of a majority of women ranges between 6 and 30 years. Only three were married for 36 to 40 years, and none beyond.

TABLE 2.9 *Distribution of women by marital duration*

| *Marital duration (in years)* | *Women* | |
|---|---|---|
| | *Number* | % |
| up to 5 | 118 | 16.55 |
| 6–10 | 119 | 16.69 |
| 11–15 | 115 | 16.13 |
| 16–20 | 88 | 12.34 |
| 21–25 | 73 | 10.24 |
| 26–30 | 118 | 16.55 |
| 31–35 | 79 | 11.08 |
| 36–40 | 3 | 0.42 |
| Total | 713 | 100.00 |

A woman's marital duration ends with her husband's death, separation, or divorce. Eighty-five per cent of women and 97% of men in Mogra are currently married. Of the 105 widowed, one divorced and one deserted women, nearly 59% lost their husbands after they crossed the age of 40, while 32% became widows between 26 and 40 years of age, and 9% before the age of 25 (see also Table 2.2).

Table 2.10 shows distribution of women by age at first childbirth. While 272 women were married before the age of 15, 36 had their first child by then. Nearly 55% of women became mothers before crossing the age of 20, 28% between 21 and 25 years, and

TABLE 2.10 *Distribution of women by age at first childbirth*

| *Age at 1st childtbirth (in years)* | *Women* | |
|---|---|---|
| | *Number* | *%* |
| Up to 15 | 36 | 5.05 |
| 16–20 | 355 | 49.79 |
| 21–25 | 196 | 27.49 |
| 26–30 | 26 | 3.65 |
| 31–35 | 4 | 0.56 |
| 36+ | 3 | 0.42 |
| Not yet mothers | 93 | 13.04 |
| Total | 713 | 100.00 |

over 4% after 25 years of age. As many as 93 (13.04%) have not attained motherhood yet (see Table 2.11 for their age distribution).

TABLE 2.11 *Distribution of childless women by age*

| *Age (in years)* | *Childless women* |
|---|---|
| 11–15 | 5 |
| 16–20 | 57 |
| 21–25 | 22 |
| 26–30 | 3 |
| 31–35 | 1 |
| 36–45 | 1 |
| 46+ | 4 |
| Total | 93 |

A majority of these 93 childless women are young brides, married for less than three years (see Table 2.12 and for contrast,

Table 2.9). Sixty-two of them are below 20. Except for nine women aged 26 and above, all others are below 25. As many as 67 of the 93 women were married between 16 and 20 years of age.

As custom restricts motherhood to married women, it is pertinent to see how many childless women are not presently married. Table 2.13 shows five women, four of whom are widowed and one

TABLE 2.12 *Childless women by marital duration*

| *Marital duration (in years)* | *Childless women* |
|---|---|
| Up to 3 | 59 |
| 4–5 | 17 |
| 6–10 | 12 |
| 11–15 | 2 |
| 16+ | 3 |
| Total | 93 |

TABLE 2.13 *Childless women by marital status*

| *Marital status* | *Childless women* |
|---|---|
| Married | 88 |
| Widowed/divorced | 5 |
| Total | 93 |

divorced. Of the remaining 88 childless women, 67 are newly married and may become mothers sooner than later, while 19 married for more than five years are hopeful of becoming mothers. Childless women will be discussed in detail in Chapter 3.

Table 2.8 shows that girls are maried at an early age in Mogra. So they become mothers-in-law at an early age (see Table 2.14). Kolenda (1989) aptly observes that it is typical in rural Rajasthan for couples in their thirties and forties to give directions to their inexperienced married teenaged sons and daughters-in-law. In a few households, the teenaged daughter-in-law is supervised by her mother-in-law as well as the latter's mother-in-law. In Mogra there are 12 such cases.

Of the 713 ever married women, 620 are mothers. Of these, 255 are mothers-in-law. Table 2.14 shows that almost 75% of the mothers-in-law attained the status before crossing the age of 40.

TABLE 2.14 *Respondents by age at mother-in-lawhood*

| *Age at mother-in-lawhood (in years)* | *Mothers-in-law* | |
|---|---|---|
| | *Number* | % |
| Up to 30 | 3 | 1.18 |
| 31–35 | 73 | 28.63 |
| 36–40 | 111 | 43.53 |
| 41–45 | 50 | 19.61 |
| 46–50 | 15 | 5.88 |
| 51–55 | 2 | 0.78 |
| 56+ | 1 | 0.39 |
| Total | 255 | 100.00 |

## *Fertility Performance of Women in Mogra*

Since 93 of 713 women are childless—88 young and not-yet-mothers, and five barren—the following data will pertain to the remaining 620 women.

Table 2.15 shows the distribution of mothers by five income groups and the number of children born to them. The 244 and 161 mothers belonging to the third and fourth income groups respectively show high fertility, while the nine and 87 mothers in the lowest and highest income groups respectively have fewer children. The modal value for the entire distribution is five children per mother. The mode in the poorest income category is 1–3 children. There are fewer mothers with 7–9 and 10 or more children, i.e., 173, compared with 230 in the 4–6 children category, and 217 in the 1–3 children category. These figures show that fertility is lower among mothers in households with the lowest and the highest incomes. The lower fertility of women in the lowest income group in Mogra is contrary to the view presented in demographic studies by Wyon and Gordon (1971) for Punjab; Chandrasekaran and George (1962) for Bengal; Gaiha (1982) for all India rural households 1968–69, 70–71, and 71–72; and Lipton (1984) for data

TABLE 2.15 *Distribution of mothers by number of children born and annual household income*

| *Income (in Rs)* | *Mothers with number of children born* | | | | | | *Mean No. of chld per mother* |
|---|---|---|---|---|---|---|---|
| | *1–3 chld* | *4–6 chld* | *7–9 chld* | *10+ chld* | *Total mothers* | *%* | |
| Up to 2,500 | 5 | 4 | 0 | 0 | 9 | 01.5 | 3.33 |
| 2,501–5,000 | 47 | 47 | 23 | 2 | 119 | 19.2 | 4.49 |
| 5,001–10,000 | 78 | 85 | 65 | 16 | 244 | 39.4 | 5.23 |
| 10,001–20,000 | 57 | 63 | 29 | 12 | 161 | 26.0 | 4.92 |
| 20,000+ | 30 | 31 | 23 | 3 | 87 | 14.0 | 4.96 |
| Total | 217 (35.0) | 230 (37.1) | 140 (22.6) | 33 (5.3) | 620 | 100.00 | 4.94 |

Note: chld = children

computed by Visaria (1980) for his study of poverty and living standards in India. On the other hand, Anker (1977) reports on the basis of a sample that low income groups from rural Gujarat have low fertility, as found in Mogra. Singh (1986) in her study of rural communities in Punjab and Haryana finds little variation in mean number of children across income groups. Jain (1975) rightly concludes that fertility differentials between different income groups in rural areas are small, especially because cultural practices, which are real determinants of fertility behaviour, do not differ with changes in income.

As income in Mogra is largely dependent on land ownership, it is necessary to relate land ownership with fertility. Table 2.16 shows this relationship. The mode is 4–6 children per mother. The landless and those with meagre patches of land (up to 2 acres) have fewer children than those with 2–5 and 6–25 acres of land. Beyond 26 acres, the number of mothers in all categories of birth decreases. At the same time there are more mothers with 10 or more children in the groups owning 6–25 acres and 26–50 acres of land. All these variations are, however, hardly significant as the mean number of children born per mother is nearly uniform for all groups. Landless couples at one end and those who own 26–50 acres of land at the other have near equal number of children.

TABLE 2.16 *Distribution of mothers by number of children born and land ownership of the household*

| *Land owned (in acres)* | *Mothers with number of children born* | | | | | | *Mean No. of chld per mother* |
|---|---|---|---|---|---|---|---|
| | *1–3 chld* | *4–6 chld* | *7–9 chld* | *10+ chld* | *Total mothers* | *%* | |
| Nil | 23 | 29 | 12 | 0 | 64 | (10.3) | 4.48 |
| 1 to 5 | 29 | 40 | 15 | 4 | 87 | (14.0) | 4.77 |
| 6 to 25 | 90 | 94 | 60 | 19 | 263 | (42.4) | 5.01 |
| 26 to 50 | 48 | 42 | 36 | 9 | 135 | (21.8) | 5.06 |
| 51+ | 27 | 26 | 17 | 1 | 71 | (11.5) | 4.67 |
| Total | 217<br>(35.0) | 230<br>(37.1) | 140<br>(22.6) | 33<br>(5.3) | 620 | <br>(100.0) | 4.94 |

Note: chld = children
unequal interval between landowning groups is primarily because of meaningful concentration of people in them.

Statistically speaking, the mean ranges from 4.48 to 5.06 for the two groups respectively. The overall mean is 4.94 children per mother. The tendency for fertility to increase with increase in land ownership reverses in the group with the largest amount of land. The distribution in Table 2.16 thus does not show any linear correlation between fertility and land ownership. Driver (1963) reports negligible difference on an average, i.e., 4.5 children for landless as against 4.6 for landowners in central India. Mamdani (1972) finds everyone wanting more children irrespective of land ownership in Khanna villages in Punjab.

There is an inverse correlation between education and fertility in Mogra (see Table 2.17). Literacy is almost non-existent among mothers. We have noted in the previous chapter that sending children, especially girls, to school is given little priority. Therefore, a very large proportion of couples, especially wives, are illiterate in Mogra—96.36% as against 57% men. Nineteen men have been to college compared with only one woman. Only 23 have ever been to school and four of these have not had any child, leaving only 19 mothers who have ever been to school. Only one out of these 19 completed high school and attended college for a

TABLE 2.17 *Distribution of women and their husbands by education*

| *Level of education* | *Women* | | *Women's husbands* | |
|---|---|---|---|---|
| | *Number* | *%* | *Number* | *%* |
| Illiterate | 687 | 96.36 | 408 | 57.22 |
| Literate | 3 | 0.42 | 56 | 7.86 |
| 1–5 years of school | 19 | 2.66 | 119 | 16.69 |
| 6–8 years of school | 1 | 0.14 | 62 | 8.70 |
| 9–11 years of school | 2 | 0.28 | 49 | 6.87 |
| 12+ years of education | 1 | 0.14 | 19 | 2.66 |
| Total | 713 | 100.00 | 713 | 100.00 |

year, two completed middle school, and one, primary school, while the rest did not even complete primary school. And this education has had little impact on fertility: 11 have 1–3 children each, seven have 4–6, and one has seven children. One of these 19 is aged above 45, while the rest are below 35, showing that education for women is a very recent phenomenon in Mogra.

Table 2.18 shows distribution of women by their husbands' education and the number of children they have had. There are as many as 194 men who have ever been to school. The proportion of illiterate husbands having more than three children (73.80%) is larger than that of their literate (those who can read and write at least their names and addresses without having been to school) counterparts (48.76%). Also, 25 of the 33 fathers with 10 or more children are illiterate. However, for a deeper understanding the data in Table 2.18 needs to be put in a proper perspective. Of the 242 fathers in the literate group, as many as 102 have been to primary school (for five years or less). Of the rest, 92 fathers have had six or more years of education, and only 17 have cleared school or entered college and/or university. Moreover, a significant limitation of Table 2.18 is that it does not reveal the fact that the educated fathers belong to a younger age group. As a school was opened in Mogra only three decades ago in 1954 and it took a few years to gain popularity even among male children, most of the educated fathers are in the age group of 20–30. Fifty-eight fathers are aged up to 25, 100 between 26–35, 27 between 36–45, and nine

TABLE 2.18 *Distribution of women by number of children born and husband's education*

| *Husband's educational level* | *Mothers with number of children born* | | | | | | *Mean No. of chld per mother* |
|---|---|---|---|---|---|---|---|
| | *1–3 chld* | *4–5 chld* | *7–9 chld* | *10+ chld* | *Total mothers* | *%* | |
| Illiterate | 99 | 146 | 108 | 25 | 378 | 61.0 | 5.46 |
| Literate | 15 | 17 | 9 | 7 | 48 | 7.7 | 5.50 |
| 1–5 years of school | 43 | 37 | 21 | 1 | 102 | 16.5 | 4.41 |
| 6–8 years of school | 25 | 13 | 1 | 0 | 39 | 6.3 | 3.15 |
| 9–11 years of school | 22 | 14 | 0 | 0 | 36 | 5.8 | 3.16 |
| 12+ years of education | 13 | 3 | 1 | 0 | 17 | 2.7 | 2.80 |
| Total | 217 (35.0) | 230 (37.1) | 140 (22.6) | 33 (5.3) | 620 | 100.0 | 4.94 |

Note: chld = children

over 45. By virtue of being younger in age most of the ever-been-to-school fathers have been married for a shorter duration. Owing to these two factors, the fertility of younger couples is slightly lower than that of the older ones irrespective of their educational status. This new trend is further discussed in Chapter 7.

In demographic literature, family type has been correlated with fertility. Some studies have shown couples in joint families having fewer children (Bebarta 1966; Poti and Dutta 1960; Pakrasi and Malaker 1967), while some others have argued that joint families have higher fertility (Mamdani 1972; Mandelbaum 1974). At any given point in time some statistical correlation is bound to exist between family type and fertility (see Table 2.19 for instance) but it may not be logical. Proportionately more women in simple households have had 4–6 and nine or more children, while more women in complex households have had 1–3 and 7–9 children. The average fertility in complex households is 4.88 children per mother, while it is 4.57 in simple households. This is hardly a significant difference.

TABLE 2.19 *Distribution of mothers by household type and number of children born*

| *Household type* | *Mothers with number of children born* | | | | | | *Mean No. of chld per Mother* |
|---|---|---|---|---|---|---|---|
| | *1–3 chld* | *4–6 chld* | *7–9 chld* | *10+ chld* | *Total mothers* | *%* | |
| Simple | 63 | 93 | 35 | 13 | 204 | 32.9 | 4.97 |
| Complex | 154 | 137 | 105 | 20 | 416 | 67.1 | 4.93 |
| Total | 217 | 230 | 140 | 33 | 620 | 100.0 | 4.94 |
| | (35.0) | (37.1) | (22.6) | (5.3) | | | |

Note: chld = children

Of the total number of mothers, a third (204) live in simple and two-thirds (416) in complex households (see Table 2.20). On the other hand, as mentioned earlier, there are 215 ever married women in simple and 498 in complex households. While simple households have one ever married couple each, most of the complex households have more than one each. Only seven complex households have one ever married woman each, three have two couples, 44 have three, 23 have four, four have five, and three have respectively six, eight and nine couples each. The seven complex households with only one ever married woman are mostly households with widows living with son's/daughter's children.

TABLE 2.20 *Women and mothers by household type*

| *Household type* | *Women* | *%* | *Mothers* | *%* |
|---|---|---|---|---|
| Simple | 215 | 30.15 | 204 | 32.91 |
| Complex | 498 | 69.85 | 416 | 67.09 |
| Total | 713 | 100.00 | 620 | 100.00 |

All through their analyses, demographers have glossed over the developmental process of the household (Fortes 1958; Shah 1973). This makes the exercise of correlating family type with fertility futile. At any given time a household may be simple, complex, or a variation thereof. If the developmental process of the household is disregarded, then it would seem that the children of a couple were all born in one household type. The analysis will not convey how many children were born before and after the change in the household structure (type) (cf. Ryder 1976 for similar views on Yucatan). Suppose two children were born to a couple while in a joint household and two in the present simple household. The question arises: where does the couple figure with relation to family type and fertility? Demographers correlating family type with fertility have employed rather uncritically the concepts of joint and nuclear family assuming that a couple has always lived either in joint or a nuclear family. They have not bothered to inquire if the couple has experienced a change of family structure (type) during their fertility career.

Table 2.20 shows that only 416 of 498 women in complex households are mothers. Of the remaining 82, barring a few, a majority are recently-married young women. Given the nature of the household developmental process, complex households have a disproportionate number of young women. As mentioned earlier, a woman usually lives in a complex household in the initial years of her married life. She attains motherhood by the time she secedes. Of the 303 mothers who have seceded, 206 did so after having 1–3 children each. They have continued to bear children, the average number born per woman being five. Thus, the family type to which a couple belongs is not significant in influencing fertility behaviour.

As we have seen, the average number of children born to a mother is five (4.94 to be statistically precise). The birth of 4–6 children is considered the social optimum (cf. Djurfeldt and Lindberg 1976: 191 for the figure for south India). The average number of children born to an ever married woman in rural India was 5.07 in 1972 and 5.09 in 1981 (Census of India 1981b, Part II Special Statement 18: 47).

Let us now see the relation between fertility and caste in Mogra. Table 2.21 presents the distribution of mothers by number of children and caste. The mean number of children born to a mother in the upper castes is identical to the village mean, i.e., 4.94; for the upper-middle castes it is 4.70, for the lower-middle castes,

TABLE 2.21 *Distribution of mothers by Caste and number of children born*

| *Caste* | *Mothers with number of children born* | | | | | *Mean No. of chld* |
|---|---|---|---|---|---|---|
| | *1–3 chld* | *4–6 chld* | *7–9 chld* | *10+ chld* | *Total chld* | |
| Upper | 20 (34) | 24 (40) | 11 (19) | 4 (7) | 59 (100) | 4.94 |
| Upper-middle | 142 (37) | 145 (38) | 81 (22) | 12 (3) | 380 (100) | 4.70 |
| Lower-middle | 29 (37) | 22 (28) | 20 (25) | 8 (10) | 79 (100) | 5.26 |
| Lower | 26 (25) | 39 (39) | 28 (27) | 9 (9) | 102 (100) | 5.58 |
| Total | 217 (35) | 230 (37) | 140 (23) | 33 (5) | 620 (100) | 4.94 |

Note: chld = children

5.2 and for the lower castes, 5.58. The mean number of children born various caste categories thus does not vary largely between them, and from the overall village mean of 4.94. The difference between the village and the highest means is 0.64 children, i.e., about one child more for every two mothers. The modal fertility for all castes except the lower-middle is 4–6 children. For the lower-middle castes it is 1–3 children, although their mean fertility is the second highest among the castes in Mogra. Three out of every four mothers have had 1–3 and 4–6 childbirths in the upper and upper-middle castes, while two in every three mothers have had 1–3 and 4–6 childbirths in the lower-middle and lower castes. Mothers with 10 or more children are proportionately highest (10%) among the lower-middle castes, followed by 9% among the lower castes, 7% among the upper castes, and the lowest (3%) among the upper-middle castes.The data in Table 2.21 shows that upper-middle castes have the lowest fertility, followed by upper, lower-middle and lower castes respectively. There is no linear correlation between caste and fertility.

Demographers have frequently tried to correlate caste and

fertility. More often, the higher castes are shown to have lower fertility than the lower castes (Chandrasekaran and George 1962; U.N. 1961; Rele 1963; Wyon and Gordon 1971). But, these studies correlate fertility with specific caste groups without taking into account the structural conditions and social norms within a caste influencing fertility behaviour. In this regard, Kolenda (1968) and Conklin (1976) rightly observe that such correlations rarely reveal any significant association. In fact, the data in Tables 2.21 and 2.22 is presented merely to reiterate the futility of correlating caste with number of children born or surviving.

The number of children born to a mother belonging to a caste does not reveal the total picture. It is only one side of the coin. We should also see child survival, as in Table 2.22. The mean number of surviving children in Mogra is four (3.89 to be precise) children per mother. While the mean number of childbirths is identical for the village and the upper castes, the mean for child survival is identical for the village and the upper-middle castes. The mean number of surviving children for the upper castes is 3.81, for the lower-middle castes 3.75, and for the lower castes 4.03 (the largest).

TABLE 2.22 *Distribution of mothers by Caste and number of surviving children*

| *Caste* | *Mothers with number of children alive* | | | | | *Mean No. of chld alive* |
|---|---|---|---|---|---|---|
| | *1–3 chld* | *4–6 chld* | *7–9 chld* | *10+ chld* | *Total chld* | |
| Upper | 29 | 24 | 4 | 1 | 58 | 3.81 |
| | (50.0) | (41.3) | (6.9) | (1.7) | (100) | |
| Upper-middle | 174 | 161 | 30 | 4 | 369 | 3.89 |
| | (47.1) | (43.6) | (8.1) | (1.1) | (100) | |
| Lower-middle | 42 | 25 | 10 | 0.0 | 77 | 3.75 |
| | (55.0) | (32.0) | (13.0) | (0.0) | (100) | |
| Lower | 49 | 37 | 15 | 1 | 102 | 4.03 |
| | (48.0) | (36.0) | (15.0) | (1.0) | (100) | |
| Total | 294 | 247 | 59 | 6 | 606 | 3.89 |
| | (48.5) | (40.7) | (9.7) | (0.9) | (100) | |

Note: chld = children

But the village mean of 3.89 children surviving per mother hardly varies between caste categories. The lower-middle castes rank the lowest (3.75), while the lower castes rank the highest (4.03). The two are equidistant (0.14) from the village mean. In the category of mothers with 10 or more surviving children, the upper-middle castes have the largest number, followed by the upper and the lower castes, both ranking second, while the lower-middle castes are not represented in this category. When Table 2.21 and 2.22 are put together, it is clear that the fertility differential between castes is only marginal and there is not much sense in pursuing this exercise any further.

Child survival is the more important dimension of fertility. Most KAP studies in India have revealed that the question about the number of children desired has been understood by respondents invariably as the number of surviving children desired. In fact, several studies have shown that it is meaningless to ask the question about the desired family size unless it is seen in the light of real experiences of the family in the process of its reproduction under a particular set of objective conditions (U.N. 1961; Poffenberger 1969; Mamdani 1972).

The distribution in Table 2.23 appears to support most demographers' view that lower the age at marriage higher the fertility. But in reality it is rather difficult to support this view. Table 2.23

TABLE 2.23 *Distribution of mothers by number of children born and age at marriage*

| *Age at marriage (in years)* | *Mothers with number of children born* | | | | | | *Mean No. of chld per mother* |
|---|---|---|---|---|---|---|---|
| | *1–3 chld* | *4–6 chld* | *7–9 chld* | *10+ chld* | *Total mothers* | *%* | |
| Up to 14 | 33 | 40 | 35 | 1 | 122 | (19.7) | 4.50 |
| 15–20 | 177 | 186 | 103 | 18 | 484 | (78.1) | 4.76 |
| 21–25 | 6 | 3 | 2 | 1 | 12 | (1.9) | 4.50 |
| 26+ | 1 | 1 | 0 | 0 | 2 | (0.3) | 3.50 |
| Total | 217 | 230 | 140 | 33 | 620 | | 4.94 |
| | (35.0) | (37.1) | (22.6) | (5.3) | | (100) | |

Note: chld = children

shows that almost all the mothers (98%) were married either before the age of 15 or between 16 and 20. Only 14 of the 620 (2.2%) mothers were married after the age of 20. The average age at marriage is nearly 16. (It may be recalled that age at marriage of girls in Rajasthan according to the 1971 and 1981 census is 15.07 and 16.09 years respectively, compared with 17.16 and 18.32 for India as a whole). Those who had been married before the age of 15 have had lower fertility than those married between 16 and 20. The average number of children born per mother in theformer group is 5.73, while among the latter it is nearly seven. On the other hand, 14 women married after the age of 20 have lower fertility, however insignificant their number may be. The correlation between age at marriage and fertility shows both positive and negative tendencies at the same time. As in Mogra, no clear relationship between age at marriage and fertility is found in Gujarat by Anker and Anker (1982).

There is a widespread assumption in demographic literature that people in rural India go on producing children as long as they can (Enke 1966; U.N. 1974; Endres 1975). By an extension of the same logic, it is argued that early marriage provides a longer duration of procreation resulting in more childbirths and vice versa (Aggarwala 1966b; Wyon and Gordon 1971; Mandelbaum 1974; Mahadevan and Sumangala 1987). But there is also the period of adolescent infertility which demographers have neglected. Adolescent sterility has to be taken into consideration especially when demographic calculations are made to correlate age at marriage with fertility. Based on a study of the reproductive development of the female, and on a few fertility studies, Mandelbaum has pointed out:

> The human female does not develop into full reproductive maturity for several years after her first menstruation. During those years there is, on an average, significantly less chance of conception than there is after the age of 19 or 20 (1974: 36)

Girls married by 14–16 years are rarely able to enter their reproductive career soon after marriage. The period of one or two years of adolescent sterility in Mogra coincides with the expected interval, of at least two years, between marriage and motherhood. The phenomenon of adolescent sterility along with institutional mechanisms regulating birth intervals explains the lower fertility of mothers married at an early age. In Mogra the average interval between marriage and motherhood for mothers married before 15 is about three years, while for those married between 16 and 20 is 2–3 years.

Given 16 years as the average age at marriage of women and 49 at menopause, a married woman can possibly have about 16 children with the observed birth interval of two years. Aggarwala (1966a) observes that in recent decades married women in India have had an average of 6.6 children during their entire reproductive career from 15 to 45 years of age. Birdsall and Jamison (1983), while making a comparison of several countries, observe the total fertility rate for Indian women to be 4.9 in 1980, nearly the same as that of women in Mogra. Only three of the 620 mothers gave birth to 14 children each, four to 13, and five to 12. These (3+4+5) 12 mothers constitute over 2% of the total. Those with 10 or more children form 4% of the total. On an average the mothers' exposure period is 18.2 years, while their actual reproductive period (between the first and last childbirth) is 12 years.

Table 2.24 shows a positive correlation between marital duration and fertility. The modal fertility is in the 4–6 children group. Only 5.3% of all mothers have had 10 or more children each. The average fertility for 80 mothers with 31 or more years of fertility exposure

TABLE 2.24 *Distribution of mothers by number of children born and marital duration*

| *Marital duration (in years)* | *Mothers with number of children born* | | | | | | *Mean No. of chld per mother* |
|---|---|---|---|---|---|---|---|
| | *1–3 chld* | *4–6 chld* | *7–9 chld* | *10+ chld* | *Total mothers* | *%* | |
| Up to 10 | 127 | 23 | 0 | 0 | 150 | 24.2 | 2.46 |
| 11–20 | 66 | 103 | 27 | 3 | 199 | 32.1 | 4.50 |
| 21–30 | 20 | 80 | 74 | 17 | 191 | 30.8 | 6.38 |
| 31+ | 4 | 24 | 39 | 13 | 80 | 12.9 | 7.28 |
| Total | 217<br>(35.0) | 230<br>(37.1) | 140<br>(22.6) | 33<br>(5.3) | 620<br>(100.0) | | 4.94 |

Note: chld = children

is seven children. In fact, four have had only 1–3 children each. The data does not support some demographers' view that rural couples procreate as long as they can. Child mortality impinges on a couple's fertility. How notions and behaviour regarding optimum fertility interact with child mortality incidences is discussed in Chapter 5.

Table 2.25 shows fertility by mother's age. Although the distribution shows that the number of children tends to increase with mother's age, most of the older mothers have had 4–6 and 7–9 children. On an average, mothers aged 36 and above have had

TABLE 2.25 *Distribution of mothers by their age and number of children born*

| *Mothers' age (in years)* | *Mothers with number of children born* | | | | | | *Mean No. of chld per mother* |
|---|---|---|---|---|---|---|---|
| | *1–3 chld* | *4–6 chld* | *7–9 chld* | *10+ chld* | *Total mothers* | % | |
| Up to 25 | 98 | 17 | 0 | 0 | 115 | 18.5 | 2.44 |
| 26–35 | 77 | 93 | 20 | 4 | 194 | 31.3 | 4.24 |
| 36–45 | 19 | 50 | 50 | 9 | 128 | 20.6 | 6.14 |
| 46+ | 23 | 70 | 70 | 20 | 183 | 29.5 | 6.42 |
| Total | 217 (35.0) | 230 (37.1) | 140 (22.6) | 33 (5.3) | 620 (100.0) | | 4.94 |

Note: chld = children

6.31 children. Of these mothers, those betwen 36 and 45 have had 6.14 children each and those above 46 years, 6.42 children each. While 20 mothers in the senior-most group have had 10 or more children each, 23 of them have had 1–3 children each. Only 2% of the senior-most mothers with completed fertility have had 10 or more children each; they thus constitute a tiny minority. Younger as well as older mothers seem to be governed by common social norms constraining the former to procreate and the latter to stop procreation. The above figures and the fact that the mean number of children born to mothers is 4.94, contradict some demographers' view that rural people reproduce as long as they can.

As seen earlier, the average age at mother-in-lawhood in Mogra is 35 years while the mode is 40. Most women prefer to stop procreating by the age of 35, while some continue for some more time for a variety of reasons to be discussed in Chapter 5. Almost a fourth of the mothers-in-law who happen to have had children (see Table 2.26) had done so much to their own chagrin. Nevertheless, they were soon able to control their situation and discontinue procreation. Fewer mothers from the upper castes than those from the other castes have had children after attaining the status of mother-in-law. This may also be explained by the higher age at marriage in this group, and consequently higher age of attaining mother-in-law status. They rarely procreate after that. Grandmothers in Mogra conform to the precepts of the village community (see Chapter 6 for an account).

TABLE 2.26 *Women by children born after mother-in-lawhood*

| *Children* | *Mothers-in-law* |
|---|---|
| 0 | 184 |
| 1 | 39 |
| 2 | 19 |
| 3 | 10 |
| 4 | 3 |
| Total | 225 |

However, some mothers-in-law do violate the norm, get pregnant and have a child or more after attaining this status. Of the 255 mothers-in-law, 71 (27.8%) have had child(ren) after their son or daughter was married. How do people react when they learn of a pregnant mother-in-law? What do other senior women prefer to do with regard to their own pregnancy? What efforts do they make to avoid pregnancy after their eldest child's marriage? These questions will be dealt with in Chapters 3, 6, and 7.

CHAPTER 3

# *Social and Cultural Context of Fertility*

Fertility behaviour includes not only biological but also social reproduction, involving a complex network of institutions. As Fortes highlights: 'The process of social reproduction, in broad terms, includes all those institutional mechanisms and customary activities and norms which serve to maintain, replenish and transmit the social capital from generation to generation' (1958: 2). Biological reproduction needs to be seen in the context of social reproduction. (see Meillassoux, 1991: 23–140 for an elaboration on this distinction in slavery, and for social context see Mac Cormack ed. 1982). Fertility behaviour, including childbirth, is the outcome of a complex web of institutional mechanisms regulated by social norms and cosmology. People's perception of fertility, and their values and attitudes are intricately interwined with social institutions. For analytical purposes, fertility behaviour is divided into domestic, economic and political spheres (cf. Srinivas and Ramaswamy 1977).

## *Domestic Sphere*

Parenthood confers honour on a couple in Mogra. A person graduates to the status of a full-fledged adult only upon acquiring parenthood. It is supposed to make individuals more responsible and trustworthy in their households and the community. It is believed to be an insignia of individual maturity and greater knowledge of the world. A person's image and respectability get enhanced with every additional child's birth and survival. A couple with four to five surviving children is held in high esteem than younger couples without children.

The consummation of marriage heralds a transformation in the woman's status. She has to take on more difficult jobs at home as well as on land (except among those castes where women observe *purdo* and do not work in fields). As a new entrant in the conjugal home, she has to work under her mother-in-law's strict supervision. It is only by becoming a mother that she can establish her common interest in the household. The mother-in-law's behaviour is generally domineering and authoritarian. The ideal daughter-in-law is one who is meek, docile and subservient. She is expected to be respectful and deferential. The relationship tends to be stress-laden, but there are few open confrontations while she is young. She has to fend for herself in the several discords that occur in the household. The young husband cannot support her. A partisan husband is critized as being henpecked.

The mother-in-law is the most effective agent in channelizing the institution of patriarchy in the household. She teaches her sons to keep their dominance over their wives and children. The daughters-in-law are not allowed to raise their voice before their husbands and other elders in the household. Daughters are often made aware, especially by the mother, that they would have to adapt to conditions in their conjugal household, thereby preparing them for a subservient role there. My encounter with two young girls aged 6–7 years reveals the extent to which the principle of subordination is inculcated at such a tender age.

> Meera and Chimu desired to see the place I was staying in. They accompanied me to it in the scorching heat of the May sun. On the way, the older of the two inquired about my household. She was surprised to hear that I lived all alone in the house. 'I would never be able to live like this', she said. The younger girl countered in an elderly tone, 'You will be thrashed if you don't do as ordered'. By implication, even young girls are prepared to orders unquestioningly. More so in their conjugal households when they grow up.

Motherhood integrates the daughter-in-law in the conjugal household. This is true of all castes but much more of those that permit *nāta*. Among the latter, a childless widow is more likely to get remarried (as discussed in Chapter 2). The chances of remarriage are less if she has children. Similarly, a young woman without children can seek separation (or divorce) more easily and get remarried. Children bind the widow emotionally to her conjugal household. Her emotional dependence on her natal home is shifted on to her children. She emerges stronger in the household as her children grow to adolescence.

Fertility ensures the mother a permanent position in the conjugal household. Childbirth lends stability and security to the bride's relationship with other household members. If a woman does not bear any child for 4–5 years after marriage there is serious concern. Also a fear that the man might bring in another wife. Motherhood is believed to transform the less adjusting bride into one more adaptable to the conjugal household. As a proverb says: 'Let her have a few children and her wings will be clipped'.

After establishing herself as a mother, a woman overcomes her disabilities as a bride and daughter-in-law and gains some authority. Inspite of graduation in status, the young mother remains subordinate in her conjugal household as long as others, especially the mother-in-law, are present. She has only a marginal say even in the marriage of her own children, especially among castes where child marriage is practised. It is common for the in-laws to arrange the wedding of her children, especially if she resides with them.

The filial bond dominates the conjugal bond in Mogra. The wife's relationship with the husband is characterized by deference, especially in the initial stge of marriage. The norms enjoin that the husband and wife have minimal interaction lest their relationship become strong enough to undermine all other relations in the household and endanger its unity. The wife is supposed to conceal familiarity with her husband during daytime. She has to cover her face with *gũngto*, or observe *purdo* and remain in the women's section of the house. Young spouses meet each other only when the rest of the household retires for the night. The young bride interacts directly and frequently with members younger to her husband, and usually does so without a *gũngto*.

It is only after several years of marriage, coupled with attainment of motherhood, that she can dare uncover her face and talk directly to the older women of the household and the neighbourhood. The veil is never removed before the elderly male in-laws. The older women strictly enforce this custom and the younger ones comply unquestioningly. Any deviance is severely criticized as lacking in modesty and decorum. It is only after having a few grown up children that a woman can interact with her husband in public. By the time she begins to interact more freely she is either a mother-in-law or some other type of senior woman in the household.

The domination of the filial over the conjugal bond is so striking that a daughter-in-law is considered an alien grafted to the conjugal household. The wife is considered to be dispensable, while it is impossible to substitute one's parents. Childbirth changes the status of a bride into that of a mother. With the passage of time her husband's younger siblings also get married. She gains seniority, as a result of which she interacts somewhat more freely with the elder women of the household, and also contemplates establishing her own simple household by seceding from the complex one. This does not require partitioning the household property. The latter is a long drawn process and usually takes place over a fairly long period after separation.

Although a strong filial bond is the ideal and separation from parents is not smooth for married sons, it does take place nevertheless. A proverb reinforces the conjugal over the fraternal bond: 'There would be as many households as brothers' (*bhāiyon jitta ghar*). Although the daughter-in-law has some role in initiating partition, she generally becomes the sole target of criticism for having begun the process of secession. The attack is softened partly if she has lived for several years in a joint household, by which time she would have a few children.

Motherhood enables a woman to be more assertive in several household affairs, including disputes. The sheer fact of having several children is indicative of a long residence in the conjugal household. This in itself is status enhancing. But mere residence does not confer status as much as motherhood does. Fertility achievements along with a long marital life, hard work and seniority in age contribute to status enhancement. Karve aptly remarks: 'It is not rare to see women who were nothing but meek non-entities blossom into positive personalities in their middle-aged widowhood or boss over the . . . old husband in the latter part of married life' (1965: 136).

### *Status of Barren Women*

Status graduation through motherhood is so marked that barrenness is a dreaded condition. The inferior status accorded to barren women is the other side of the high value accorded to fertility. Motherhood is extolled, while barrenness is held as a curse. If a woman does not produce children, her husband has the prerogative to divorce her or marry another. Sterility spells social and emotional doom for the woman. She is considered an ill omen both for the household and the larger society. It is inauspicious to run into her early in the morning or on auspicious occasions, such as rituals of childbirth, wedding and marriage, or while setting out of the house to the fields for sowing, or to another village or city. These considerations are indicative of her lower status. In quarrels and squabbles she is insulted for her failure in fertility performance. The dart of barrenness is thrown at her to whittle down her strength and to latently glorify fertility. She is under constant pressure from household members, relatives and neighbours to produce children.

In a male-dominated society a barren woman's status gets further lowered as it is always her fecundity that is doubted. Rarely is male fertility questioned. Men are rarely expected to undergo fecundity tests, while a few women have been made to do so when they did not bear any children for several years after marriage. Indigenous medication is adopted invariably by such women to be able to procreate and overcome the stigma. If a woman does not have any child after 5–6 years of marriage, she feels persuaded to explore indigenous medicines thought to help procreation. These are procured through relatives, friends, *dais* (midwives) and priests. Various rituals are observed and vows made to family and local deities. Visits to *thān* (spirit centres) are made to seek a solution to infertility. A few women who have had only one child each despite several years of marriage, have been occasionally visiting a *thān* about 40 kms from Mogra for several years. Most of them claim to have been blessed by the spirit of that *thān*. The restlessness and fear experienced by the childless women is a response to the oppressive treatment meted out to the barren. This does not mean that childless men do not face similar humiliation. Their position though is not as stigmatized as that of barren women.

Not all childless women, however, have had to face divorce or the trauma of their husband's second marriage. Second marriage is less common because bride price makes a second wife very expensive in most castes. Moreover, childlessness is not always a result of barrenness. It could result from infant and child mortality. Similarly, the absence of a male child does not evoke the stigma of barrenness. There is also the uncertainty of childbirth and child survival in a second marriage. Cases of infant mortality and deaths of adult children are usually recalled to offset divorce or remarriage plans.

A barren woman usually fights a losing battle. She faces innuendoes during quarrels and disputes.

> Cuki, 26-year-old Patel woman, was constantly worried about her childlessness despite 11 years of marriage. Her husband was losing hope in her fecundity. Her mother was equally anxious and felt awkward at social gatherings, births and other occasions, especially when people inquired of any good news of Cuki's procreation. Once during a quarrel with a neighbouring woman, Cuki felt crushed on being reminded of her infertility. She was told, 'You are barren. No one wants to even see your face.'
>
> Anadi, a 25-year-old potter woman maried for 11 years, faced a great deal of humiliation from her husband's brothers' wives. They were against her getting an equal share of the joint family property for being barren.
>
> Phool, a 28-year-old barber woman married for 12 years, always engaged herself in activities that distracted her from the regular unpleasant reminders of infertility. She either spent time in a temple run by a Charan widow, called Satiji, or went to school to be with teachers. She was rarely found at home during most of the day. 'What is the use of sitting with women in the neighbourhood? They only talk of children. I prefer to avoid an awkward situation. In the temple they are somewhat restrained', Phool surmized.
>
> Satiji is a young Charan childless widow who lost her husband within two months of mariage. Women among Charans and Rajputs have a long tradition of sacrifice and even fatal self-denial. While a widow's self-immolation on the deceased husband's pyre is a well-known form of sati, renouncing the world upon widowhood is

> another form which is locally called *jīvat sati*, or literally, living *sati*. Another Charan widow, Durga, who lives in Mogra (her natal village), is in her fifties. She had no children during the five years of her marriage. Upon widowhood, she decided against living in her conjugal household. That would have entailed numerous restraints. As a widow she was entitled to receive maintenance from the conjugal property. She thus joined her father and stepmother in her natal home after convincing her in-laws about her decision. There was little to occupy her in the conjugal household.

Unlike Durga, widows with children continue to live in their conjugal households. Their motherhood provides them the respectful status and emotional mooring not available to childless widows. Fertility and household work are the two major domains of Charan women. They face the maximum threat of divorce in the event of sterility.

> Rekha, a Charan mother, was verbally threatened by her husband when she did not bear any child for seven years after marriage. Phatu, a Charan *patwari* (village accountant) in his thirties, has had no child even after more than 12 years of marriage. His wife is perpetually anxious about her future. Her husband's second marriage is a constant fear.

In all, there are five barren women (i.e., without a child till the age of 40 years) apart from the Charan widows, Durga and Satiji, mentioned above. Of these two women, a Daroga and a Patel, are widows. The other two, a Patel and a Bhambi, are currently married. The fifth a Patel widow, was divorced by her husband for being childless for several years after marriage. She was the second wife to be divorced by the same man for barrenness. She lives with her brother's only son. However, the man's third wife also did not bear any child. She is one of the two barren widows in Mogra. She has adopted her deceased husband's brother's son, who willingly joined her to inherit her large property. The following case highlights how a barren woman may have to accept a co-wife.

> Labu, a Bhambi, is one of the two currently married barren women. She is the first of two wives of her husband. As she did not bear a child despite several years of marriage, she went along with her husband's decison to have a second wife with a view to having children. The second wife, Kanwari was blind. Labu looked after her. Kanwari had three sons, who were brought up by Labu. Despite being blind, Kanwari has been cared for respectfully by

her barren co-wife. She has greater authority in the family despite being the junior wife. The three parents live with one son each in three different houses adjacent to one another.

Labu's case shows that Harijans share the same values as other castes, especially in the stigma attached to barrenness, and the importance of a son. They enter into polygynous unions, adopt sons, or bring in *ghar jamāis* in the event of childlessness. When the assumed-to-be barren woman's pregnancy is first noticed, her status in the household and the community improves immediately. Two such cases may be recalled here:

> During my fieldwork, Cuki had a son and Anadi was in an advanced stage of pregnancy. Cuki's childbirth silenced her husband's sisters and his brothers' wives. On a later visit to the field, I learnt that the birth of Anadi's daughter had made her quite confident in the family. Both Cuki and Anadi gained self-esteem as the stigma of barrenness was erased.

### *Virtues of Parenthood*

The birth of a child to young childless couples, particularly those married for about three years is eagerly awaited by the household, other relatives, and neighbours. Childbirth dispels immediately the stigma of barrenness of a couple, especially the wife. As a first child even a daughter is welcome, although a son is more so. This is because a couple's fertility is on test. So the child's sex is secondary. Upon the first childbirth, people generally inquire first about the health of the mother and the infant, and then about the latter's sex. A successful child delivery is desirable. At this stage, the child's sex is not very important. If the first child is a girl, people frequently comment, 'She will bring a brother next time (*hamkē bhāi lāi*),' and 'Those who have a daughter will have sons too (*bēti vae toe bēta ee vēi*).' A daughter is called 'curd' and a son 'milk', and it is considered ideal for a household to have both milk and curd.

A daughter provides a great deal of help to her parents in household and other tasks before she is married. Even after marriage, she does a lot of work in her natal home whenever she visits it. As discussed briefly in Chapters 1 and 2, among castes practising the institution of *ghar jamāi*, a daughter's worth is nearly equal to, though not the same as, that of a son.

A daughter has considerable emotional value for her parents, especially in their old age. She is well-known for sharing with her old parents', especially her mother's, unhappiness and worries. On the other hand, a son is known to be less caring about his parent's emotional needs. A common saying about a daughter's emotional value is: '*Bēti veh toe man ree vāt ee kare, nee toe man ree man mein ee reh*' (literally, if there is a daughter one can at least share one's inner feelings, without a daughter the feelings cannot be let out). During unpleasant quarrels and rifts in the household, a married daughter or sister is usually acceptable as a neutral arbiter to almost all the members. In actual practice, married daughters play this tactful role rather successfully. A daughterless mother is pitied for having missed the luxury of enjoying a daughter's company. Parents without a daughter are also deprived of earning *punya* by spending on her and giving her away in marriage. In Mogra, a daughter's birth is not an unmitigated evil, spelling disaster on the household. Although the son is valued more than the daughter, the birth of at least one daughter is considered ideal for every married couple.

With the birth and growth of grandchildren the grandparents' status gets enhanced in society. They are held as respectable elders and guardians of large households. Grandparents play an important role in deciding the betrothals of their grandchildren. Their opinion matters in the observance of rituals and in their grandchildren's matchmaking. Couples with only a few children and no grandchildren are deprived of such socially significant roles and consequent status. The time spent in social relations and pursuit of leisure increases as children grow up and take over most of the chores. This depends primarily on one's fertility performance rather than on age. The following cases vividly portray the contrast in parental and grandparental status in relation to fertility and age.

> Maganji, a Jat in his forties, has five daughters and one son who is the youngest. Two of his daughters are married. Maganji once compared himself with one of his daughter's father-in-law. The latter has three sons and two daughters. His two sons are his first two children. Maganji commented: 'I am at least five years older than him. But he has become a *bapu* (a respectable term for an old man) so early in life because he has grown up married sons and daughters-in-law to work for him. His usual pastime is to relax at the street corner or in the village elders' meetings where he is lost

> under the influence of opium. He doesn't worry at all about running the household. My son is still young and unmarried. I am considered younger than him. It is his good luck.'

Mere age is not sufficient for a feeling of well-being. Grown up married children especially sons, are a sure way to a relaxed old age.

> Rajuji, a skinny old Patel in his late sixties, was generally reserved in interaction with fellow villagers as well as outsiders. Once I saw him holding his two-year-old daughter in one arm and carrying an empty pitcher in the other. He was walking towards the village pond to fetch water and also herding his cattle for watering them. The sight of an old man fetching water is rare. Although it is not uncommon for old men to be with small children, particularly their grandchildren. Rajuji was forced into work that was unusual for his age—carrying his own daughter, fetching water and herding cattle. He had to do it, as his wife was ailing and there was no one else in the household to relieve him. Rajuji had spent his entire life aspiring for a son. He married thrice. Two of his earlier wives died without a son. The second bore a girl who has been married off. The third wife had also borne a girl who was two years old (This was the one he was carrying.). Rajuji's was the only Patel household without any gold and silver jewellery—the most sought after security plank after land. On being asked if he expected any girl or boy from his lineage (because they would also be his immediate neighbours) to fetch water, he responded with a bland expression: 'Who will come to help me? Even friends and relatives cease to exist when needed by a lonely person. They come only when they know that the help will be reciprocated.'

Rajuji's house would have been full of people had he a few sons. He would have hardly needed outside help. His sons, daughters-in-law and grandchildren would not have let him work so hard. In fact, with a large family, others would have readily lent a helping hand, and he too would have conveniently reciprocated through his sons, their wives and children. People would have come to him on numerous ritual and festive occasions pertaining to his children's and grandchildren's life cycle events. But Rajuji's house wore a desolate look. Even one son would have made a great difference, as would a *ghar jamāi*. But Rajuji had given it little thought because he was hopeful of a son from every new wife after the death of the earlier one.

> Bansoji, an untouchable in his forties, lamented: 'What is there in

> life for us? Though I am pretty old, I don't have grown up children. Only this three-year-old girl is alive out of the nine children we had. Every morning we get ready for work. She (his wife) does not keep well and has to stay at home sometimes. My three younger brothers have grown up children who help their parents to earn money, graze goats and fetch water and fuel. On the other hand, we have to purchase milk for this girl. A few more children and this would have been a different household. All my brothers' children are engaged. They receive numerous guests. Their houses are full of life all the time, while we have only this little girl to talk to. I feel depressed and do not wish to meet my brothers' guests.'

Childlessness or death of several children pushes parents into a perpetual state of despair. They lose hope in life and turn indifferent to people and events around them. They prefer a general withdrawal from the wider community, unlike those with a few grown up children.

### *Social Onomastics*

The fertility norm is reinforced by various cultural practices and symbolic expressions. The institution of personal nomenclature is an important case in point. Names are not mere labels to identify and address people, but also suggest some of the significant aspects of social structure. Social onomastics in Mogra reinforces ideas about the desirability or otherwise of childbirth during certain stages in a couple's fertility trajectory.

As fertility is not a concern solely of the couple, children, especially the first few, are rarely named by young parents.[1] The first child gets its name from the mother's natal home where she goes for the first confinement. The next child is named by the father's kin. Parents have an opportunity to name their third or fourth child when grandparents attend to their other children's offspring, and parents have greater authority over their own. Naming is generally done without much ritual and ceremony.

[1] The Brahmin priests, while preparing a child's horoscope, suggest a few syllables that form the first syllables of a child's name. But this practice is prevalent only among the upper castes. Among other castes only the well off prefer to avail such a luxury. Horoscopes are generally prepared for boys, and rarely for girls even among the upper castes.

It is usually possible to decipher from the child's name the particular stage of the parents' fertility trajectory. Certain names are prescribed or preferred for the first few children, while certain others are proscribed. Another set of names is usually meant only for children born after the couple's fertility expectations are met. A few of the preferred names for the first few desired children are Asa or Asi (hope), Rana (king), Rani (queen), Sukhi (well-being), and names of deities such as Ram and Sita. Other names mean vegetation, courage, undefeated, immovable, magnanimous, wealth, jewels and immortal. As the first few children glorify the parents' status, their names are chosen accordingly. The child's position in the parents' fertility career itself rules out certain names and leaves open the possibility of certain others. The pool of preferred names may be divided into three categories—one, indicating desire for children, the other, anxiety about the child's survival, and a third, suggesting the undesirability of children. In the present chapter we have discussed the first category of names. The other two shall be discussed in Chapters 5 and 6 respectively.

### *Husband-Wife Communication*

Frequently, in demographic literature, lack of communication between spouses is reported to enhance fertility and minimize its control. For instance, Poffenberger (1969) has elaborately described the lack of communication between spouses in traditional families in Gujarat. He observes that there is least communication when the spouses are young, especially while living in joint households. On the other hand, those in nuclear households communicate more and have fewer children than those in joint households.

In Mogra, the relationship between inter-spousal communication and fertility is not so clear. Communication between young spouses in joint households is minimal. Most young couples tend to live in joint households owing to the prevalence of adolescent marriages (see Kolenda 1989 for elaboration of this feature in rural Rajasthan). Logically, couples in nuclear households do communicate with each other more, which therefore should tend to suppress fertility and maximize its control. However, in Mogra, couples seceding from joint households within one or two years of marriage tend to have as many children as those living longer in, or not seceding from, joint households. Almost all seceding couples live within the same house or on the same street. So their interaction with the patrikin and neighbours continues. The influence of even geographically distanced older relatives on the fertility of couples residing in nuclear households in Karnataka is reported by Ramu (1988: 154).

Apart from overlooking the influence of relatives on couples in nuclear households, Poffenberger's view does not recognize sufficiently the influence of the developmental process of the household. Couples are expected to have a few children in the initial stages of the developmental process (see Chapter 4), and to stop having them once the socially optimum number is achieved (see Chapter 6). It so happens that the newly-married couple's residence in a joint household and minimal communication between them during this phase coincide with their initiation into the fertility career. The deveopmental process of the household on the one hand and the beginning of the young couple's fertility career on the other are more closely related to fertility outcomes than the lack of communication between spouses.

While commenting on the relationship between lack of inter-spousal communication and high fertility, Poffenberger has probably in mind an implicit model of couples practising low fertility in a highly modernized society. Srinivas and Ramaswamy (1977: 10) rightly observe that couples are not free agents, i.e., they are not absolutely free to design their own fertility course. The assumption that couples are all free is simplistic.

Dialogue constantly takes place between the individual and the larger community. For a couple in Mogra the fertility career is charted by the norms of wider society. This should not however, mean that couples follow the norms mechanically. They know the permissible range within which their fertility behaviour can vary. They know when the number of children is less or more than required, and what their optimum number and sex composition should be.

The new entrant to the reproductive career is aware of prevailing norms, precepts and practices. Even young unmarried children know the fertility norms and react with surprise if others' fertility performance falls short of the customary expecation.

> Buddha, a 13-year-old Patel boy, was inquistive about the number of children I had. He asked my 12-year-old daughter, as to how many brothers and sisters she had. On hearing that she had only one brother he responded with surprise, 'Oh no! you should have one more brother. Your parents must have at least one more son. One son is no son just as one eye is no eye (*ēk ank mein ānk nee, ne ēk pūt mein pūt nee*).'
>
> I lived all by myself during the initial stage of fieldwork. A Patel lady next door introduced me to Hanuman, her six-year-old son who was inquisitive about me. The boy looked around for sometime and whispered to his mother. He was asking her: 'But where are her children?'

Even small children failed to understand the independence and individuality of an adult female. A woman without in-laws or children around is a deviant from the norm in their perception.

Children in Mogra are occasional witnesses to the reproductive processes of cattle and other animals. Teenaged boys and girls also learn about sexual behaviour through their peer groups. However, married and unmarried adolescent children rarely discuss such matters with elderly relatives and parents. This inhibition persists even in the initial years of marriage, when couples are aware that sexual intercourse is expected. The initial hesitation is overcome only with the passage of time.

> Keli once discussed her problem of having to bear undesired children with a lady doctor. She did not want any more children, having borne four sons and two daughters. After rejecting all the doctor's suggestions, and not being able to get the desired contraceptive injection, Keli said: 'The doctor (an unwed lady) was too shameless and immodest to have discussed so clearly and openly about such things. She is still unmarried. How could she then speak about such things without the slightest hesitation?'

A few years of married life, preferably with a child, provides a license to women in Mogra to talk freely about sexual matters. Younger women before attaining motherhood rarely enter into such discussions as a sign of modesty.

Traditionally expected inhibitions and the value associated with modesty render it difficult for parents to frankly discuss sex and childbirth with their newly-married adolescent child. Parents are able to talk about such matters freely to him/her only after the latter has had at least one child or been married for several years.

On asking whether they communicate with their spouses regarding sex and childbirth, I got a response that the adolescent typically give to the elderly. Young married girls generally bowed their heads and lowered their eyes as a sign of embarrassment and inhibition. The usual responses I got were: 'I don't know. How do I know? What is there to know (in this matter)? What can I say?' The less evasive responses included: 'We don't talk about this. You are embarrassing me. We will not do anything extraordinary. What happens to others will happen to us too.'

Adolescents follow what Bernstein (1977) calls 'restricted code' rather than 'elaborate code' (see also Gidden's 1984 terms, 'discursive' and 'practical consciousness'). Even in later life, few spouses discuss with one another their sexual lives extensively, although other personal, social and children's issues frequently are.

### *Women's Gainful Employment*

Gainful employment of women is reported to curtail fertility (U.N. 1961; Mandelbaum 1974; Engels 1884; Papanek 1973). These stuides show an inverse relation between higher status of women, accruing from gainful activity, and fertility. They argue that once women are gainfully employed, i.e., are able to produce goods worth exchange value, or earn cash income through productive work, their status generally improves. However, status depends on how the community ranks a person as well as on how the person perceives one's own status. In fact, status needs to be seen in the context of a given society.

The problem with the concept of status of women as used in demographic studies is that it is borrowed from urban-industrial societies and then applied to rural societies to arrive at an index of women's status. The resultant conclusion is that women have low status. Status gets enhanced by the acquisition of attributes signifying high value in the socio-cultural context of a given community. Status is thus not a static category. In Mogra, a woman's status keeps evolving with the developmental processes of progression and regression of the household. With changes in household membership, there are changes in the nature of positions and relationships. A woman's status in Mogra improves with marriage, fertility, age and seniority in the household.

Women's contribution to household subsistence does not automatically lead to their status elevation. As Patel has observed: 'Contribution to the family subsistence and improvement in status are mediated by a complex dialectics of patriarchal values and women's real life experiences (1987: 126)'. Motherhood is crucial for a woman's status enhancement. Afshar's (1985) and Kabeer's (1985) studies in Iran and Bangladesh respectively support the foregoing observation.

> Chandarki, a young Patel woman in her early twenties and mother of a son and daughter once had a serious quarrel with her husband, while I and a few other people were present. He threatened to beat and drive her out of the house. At this she retorted, addressing especially the standers-by: 'Don't think that I am a sonless woman. I will bring up my son in my natal home. When he grows up I will fearlessly come back to the village with all authority. I will approach all the village elders to listen to my plight and then claim a share of this household's property for my son. Then I will live with my son on this man's (her husband's) property and constantly embarrass him. Only then will he realize that he had committed a blunder.'
>
> Heerani, a Charan woman in her forties, was deserted by her husband after he married another. For several years she lived a miserable life. She had to do away with the Charan custom of *purdo* and work in the fields, collect fuel and fetch water for herself and the children. She had two sons and as many daughters. Fortunately for her, her husband's second wife had only one daughter. When Heerani's sons grew up and took charge of the household, she pronounced with covert pride: 'He (the husband) will have to come back to me in the end. His name will be kept by my sons. When he is unable to stand on his own, his daughter will be in her conjugal home and his wife will be too weak to take his care. How long can he neglect me?'

A grown up son is considered strong enough to reclaim his deserted mother's property rights and honour. He is her protector and provider in old age. He is the one who ultimately comes to her rescue in adversity. His existence itself is a source of moral support to her.

Fertility plays a crucial role in a mother's status enhancement. The fusion of her identity with that of her conjugal household and its interest, her prolonged residence and the survival and growth of a few children, form the most significant ground for status enhancement. Also, as we shall see in Chapters 6 and 7, for consequent ability to stop bearing more children.

### *Impact of Education*

Our discussion on women's as well as men's education in Chapter 2 (see Table 2.18) shows that the bearing education has on fertility is not significant. The educated fathers' exposure to the problem of population through their middle school curricula, has had little impact on them.

The social studies text-book for Class 7 (RRPM 1984a) has three chapters devoted to population. One of them deals with the relation between population and minimum needs (food, clothing, housing education, and medicine). The chapter talks about inadequate resources and suggests population control. The chapters on Indian and world population show population growth trends and the pressure of population on insufficient resources. Information is given about less populated advanced countries with higher levels of living to show the need for population control in India. The chapter on India's population appeals that the facilities for family planning provided by the central and the Rajasthan government should be availed by all.

The social studies text-book for Class 8 (RRPM 1984b) has three chapters directly dealing with population growth and resultant problems. Two other chapters deal, rather indirectly, with the undesirable growth of population. These pertain to social and other problems of India. The geography text-book for Class 8 (RRPM 1984c) has one chapter on population and culture. All these text-books raise the issue of population outrunning resources, suggest population control, and inform that counselling for population control is available at family welfare clinics and health centres.

Fathers who have been to college and now hold urban jobs (*naukri*) are not strikingly different in their fertility behaviour from their counterparts in the village. In all there are 79 men holding *naukri*. Of them, eight have never been to school. Of these four are illiterate having two, five, five and seven children respectively. The remaining four are literate, three with two, two and seven children respectively, and one is childless. Thus only 71 of the *naukri*-holders have ever been to school, and three of them have no children. Of the 68 educated fathers with *naukri*, 39 have 1–3 children, 26 have 4–6 and three have 7–9 children. The pattern in Mogra is similar to that reported by Caldwell (1982) for non-agricultural urban conditions in Ibadan, where high fertility was considered rational. Whether the educated *naukri*-holders are identical with their illiterate counterparts in their fertility behaviour is discussed in Chapter 7.

### *Economic Sphere*

We have already discussed the contribution of adults and children to the household economy in Chapter 1. Here we shall see how their contribution and fertility behaviour are interdependent. A daughter-in-law hardly has any respite from long working hours. She is not expected to take time off for relaxing as long as there is work in the house or on the fields. There is hardly an end to her work, both in the peak agricultural and slack seasons. Nursing and caring for the infant enables her to get some relief from back-breaking tasks. I must hasten to add that a mother not only gets relief from work by looking after her baby, she also enjoys caring for it. Besides, it is common knowledge that a baby's mother does not do as much work as other women because she has to attend to it intermittently.

Childbirth brings to the mother an immediate short-term relief from work. She expects some help when the eldest child reaches six or seven years of age. A mother often comments; 'The child is growing up and will tomorrow (in the near future) get me a glass of water (symbolic of being looked after)'. A mother with a few children to help her in minding younger children and doing other small chores gradually becomes assertive in the household. Her dependence on other members of the household gets relatively reduced. On the other hand, other household members also receive help from her children and thereby depend on them for minor comforts. This enhances her as well as her husband's status both in and outside the household. A mother's interest both in physical and symbolic terms lies in having a few helping children around.

The need for more working hands is felt particularly by small households in rural India. Mamdani (1972) and Caldwell (1982: 96–8) show that variations in fertility determine which families can take advantage of economic opportunities requiring increased family labour inputs. People in Mogra are clear about the value of family labour.

> Maggi, a mother of four children, remarked: 'It was difficult for me to manage all the work when I had only two small daughters. Now my daughters help me do household work, take care of cattle, and mind the two little ones (their younger siblings). Everything will be set right when my children grow up and begin helping me on land as well. We can then cultivate more land and grow more grain.'

The arrival of a daughter-in-law is a boon to working hands in a simple household. As already mentioned, people prefer family labour to wage labour. With family labour one can avoid paying cash wages and the constant haggling with hired workers. A common saying is that agriculture can prosper only under the personal care of the field owner (*khēti dhaṇiyon chēti*). There is, however, a paradox in some people's attitude towards parents having only one surviving son. On the one hand such parents are envied because a single son keeps the household land intact, while on the other, according to society's collective experience, there is a fear that a lone son might be lost.

### *Child Rearing Practices*

Child rearing in Mogra involves minimal monetary expenses compared to a modern middle class family. (The minimal cash expenditure involved in conducting child delivery is discussed in the next chapter.) After childbirth, there are hardly any commodities to be purchased from the market for the baby. Soaps, oils, talcs, towels, diapers and other modern toilet articles are unknown. The baby is bathed in warm water, and wiped and wrapped in soft rags. Proper clothing is provided after a few days of birth. Old soft pieces of cloth are used as napkins. No special bed is purchased for the baby. Its layette is made of rags. When the baby is 4–5 months old it is put in a *ghoḍi* (cradle), a swing made of cloth hanging from a four-legged wooden stand. A broad-based basket (*dāli*) is also used as a cradle. It is hung from a branch in the field or from a beam in the house. Massaging and bathing of infants is scarcely done everyday even during summer, let alone in winter. The baby's face and hands are sponged and some oil or ghee is applied to keep flies off. The baby's bed smells of ghee, oil, milk, urine, etc., and not of perfumed toilet articles. The concept of hygiene and cleanliness is strikingly different from that of the urban middle class. Infants are usually confined to their beds and to their mothers for the first few months. The mother generally looks after the baby's physical needs, and is often helped by an elderly woman in the household.

Breast milk is the only feed for an infant till the age of 6–7 months. There are no hassles or expenses involved in arranging for milk bottles, sterilizing them, preparing the feed, etc. Although frequent bathing and changing of baby clothing is rare, breast feed provides resistance against infection and ailments. Toilet training is neither elaborate nor strict. Most children are opiated to sleep for longer durations.[2] It is also believed that opium constipates the infant and thus relieves the mother from frequently cleaning soiled napkins.

An infant's expressive and instrumental needs are looked after more by its numerous relative than by its parents alone. If the child is taken ill, other household members take care of medication. The father usually conceals his affection and other emotions towards his baby when elders are present. He refers to or addresses his child rather impersonally as 'the boy' or 'the girl' and rarely by its name before elders. Even younger mothers are criticized if they fondle the infant openly. They are expected only to look after the child's physical needs while others are there to take care of emotional needs. Parents rarely purchase clothes for the infant. They mostly come as gift from the maternal and other relatives. If a father buys clothes or shows obvious fondness for the infant, it is frowned upon or disapproved by his family and neighbours. The family, kin and neighbours contribute in their own ways towards bringing up children. For proper growth of children,

---

[2] Opium is an important element in of traditional culture of this part of Rajasthan. It is a significant constituent item of almost all ritual and ceremonial occasions. Opium is offered commonly to visitors and guests. Sharing of opium indicates mutual honour both for the host and the guest. Opium is found commonly with elderly men in Mogra. By the age of 40, most men become opium addicts. They take granules of opium with water and tea. As it is believed to be tranquilizing and constipating, it is administered for diarrhoea. An infant is given opium usually to prolong its sleep and reduce bowel movement, because opium is believed to be constipating and euphoric. This relieves the mother for other chores without having constantly to care for the infant.

a family's relations with kin and neighbours are valuable. Expenses on relatives and neighbours are therefore valued highly.

The above institutions whereby the network of relatives and neighbours contribute economically and socially towards child rearing minimize the effort and cost of child rearing, especially for an infant's parents. It is relevant to recall the micro-economic analysis of fertility in terms of costs and benefits of children. The 'choice between a baby or a car' is redundant in societies like Mogra, where the very meaning of costs and benefits is not limited to economic considerations alone.

The child is brought up on resources that are seldom provided by the parents alone. People do not calculate their household expenditure in isolation from those required for bearing and rearing of children. All expenses are viewed as household expenses. The members of a household share some of their resources with those of others, especially their kin, affines and neighbours through customary gifts, etc. The household produce is also shared by several members of the eco-system, be they relatives, priests, servants, scavengers, birds, animals, ants and other insects. Economic expenses incurred by a household on child rearing are an infinitesimal part of the total.

Members of all except the untouchable castes offer grain or flour, called (*āka*), as alms to several members of the Saad, Saami and Brahmin castes every morning. In addition, alms are given to untouchables on religious occasions. Alms-giving is perceived as a religious act bringing *punna*. It is common for a child or an aged person from each household, early in the morning, to give *āka* (a few fistfuls of grains) to sparrows, pigeons, peafowl and other birds. At times, a bowl of water is placed in the courtyard, cattle-shed and such other open places for birds. Occasionally sweetened grains and water are kept around anthills for ants. A small *hogro* (bread) is given daily to a dog or a cow. People consider such deeds a part of religious activity. Several of them reported these acts to explain their interest in religion. They thought it rather fortunate to be able to give alms even if they had to do so by cutting down their own consumption of delicacies. As distinguished from the consumption attitudes of the urban middle class, the people of Mogra consider enjoyment of delicacies and comforts by saving on the obligatory alms as base and selfish for a human being. One's actual fate is believed to rest with alms given and other acts of *punna* performed in this life.

Whenever a peasant steps into the field for sowing, he prays for a harvest sufficient not only for his household but also for the priestly castes, Harijans, birds, cattle, ants, etc. It is believed that the household produce depends on the fate (*bhāg*) of all the living beings listed above. The peasant does not reap a crop from his fate as a single individual. He 'reaps through sharing others' fate, and so should he distribute', goes the maxim. In such a social and cultural framework, an individual cannot augment his resources by putting a stop to an additional childbirth nor does he think in terms of such a calculus.

A household's spending on daily alms is sufficient to cater to the daily monetary requirement of bringing up a baby. Or a few months of alms are enough to buy one of the herbal contraceptives (discussed in Chapter 6). But an individual's withdrawal from the routine of giving alms is equated to inviting impending doom for the household. It is believed that *punna* must be earned as long as there are grains in the house.

Expenses on children and the returns from them are subjective perceptions of people. In their cosmology related to income, expenditure, consumption and work a simple calculation of cost and benefit does not find any expression. People do not think in terms of 'a baby or a car'. The attitude towards children and consumer goods is entirely different. A child is not seen as a choice made against some consumer durable. An attmept to evaluate fertility behaviour in the village in terms of such a choice is both absurd and irrelevant. The tendency to superimpose a modern consumerist instrumentality on the subjective choices of a typical villager is widespread among demographers of the micro-economic genre, like Becker (1960) and Easterlin (1975).

Parents in Mogra usually have expectations from their children pertaining to their adult productive roles. Unlike urban middle class parents' aspirations that their children be smart and healthy babies, outstanding students in school and college, and prestigious job holders in adulthood, the aspirations of parents in Mogra are different. Most of them wish that their infants survive, provide a helping hand as children, settle down as socially-influential married persons with children, and give respect to and take care of their old parents. This precludes a perception of the future as the domain of a plurality of possibilities.[3] The various stages in a child's life are seen to be largely given, so that all children born have some place in the world. Nevertheless, parents do aspire that at least one of their sons hold a white collar job. In fact, it is believed that with a few children to help parents, at least one son can be spared for education. However, not producing a child in order to save resources for the betterment of the family's future is seldom a part of the parents' survival calculus.

The values attributed to children and the social and symbolic returns that accrue to their parents are supportive of high fertility. The following is the only exceptional case which conveys the predicament of a mother with a single son, and highlights the need for several children for reasons other than mere economic ones.

> Parti, in her forties, belongs to the Tailor caste, and is well-known for providing secret assistance in fertility control. She has set up an example to others by having only one child, a son. But now, Parti sometimes wonders whether she was wise in doing so. During one of my visits to her house, she wept bitterly that her son had failed in Class 10 and then again in Class 11. Her husband, a school teacher, had explained to her that their son could not be trained for a teacher's job with such poor performance. She lamented: 'I had thought he would study well and get a *naukri* (and associated prestige). But now what will happen of us? All our hopes were vested in him. They are now shattered. I can at least unburden my grief before you, but he (her husband) cannot even cry out his heart to anyone. If only I had another son I would have consoled myself that one of them might study well and get a *naukri*. My life has been wasted thoroughly. The *sarpanch's* (Mogra's panchayat head) son passed in Class 10 in the first attempt. His wife was boasting about her son's success to me. If only I had another son who studied well, I wouldn't have been a silent listener to that woman's bragging.'

---

[3] Krause (1980) analyses the American experiment of public education for urban middle class and ghetto children. He observes how achievement becomes a cherished value for a middle class child and for middle class parents, while ghetto children depend on their usual fate.

The failure of her only son in the public examination was enough of a jolt to Parti. It signalled a less radiant future for the family. Her long standing wisdom of deliberately having one son was now under challenge. Like others in the village she began to feel that having only one son was not enough.

If only Parti had more sons, at least one of them might have achieved success in the educational sphere and got a prestigious job to further enhance the household status, while the others could have taken up tailoring, that being their traditional calling. Though *naukri* is an economic proposition, it provides social prestige and symbolic value which the wealthy Parti longed for.

It is commonly argued that only when there are three or more sons can one of them be spared for education with the hope of *naukri* after studies. Though formal education is believed to help obtain salaried jobs, parents realize that education is a relatively poor means to securing an urban job. They also find their children dropping out of school or college and remaining unemployed as well as unfit for strenuous agricultural tasks. Returns from agriculture are low. As a result of such uncertainties tension prevails in people's mind. Two sons are held as the minimum, but sterilization is seldom an option just after that. The survival of two sons and a daughter offers some assurance about future life. This assurance comes only with the birth of four or five children—the traditionally prescribed and practised average. It is at this juncture that people wish to put a stop to their fertility.

### *Political Sphere*

Most political activities of the villagers are usually centered on the village. Only occasionally do these extend beyond the village to the *chautāḷo*, *tehsil* and the district. Extra-village politics is influenced by intra-village politics. More men than women are interested in politics at the wider level. For the villagers, the village is the place where they perform most of their roles pertaining to the routine of economic and social life. Their relations with neighbourhood, lineage and *jati* members are of particular political importance. Struggles for precedence and dominance are endemic in village India (Bailey 1957; Lewis 1958; Mandelbaum 1970 and many others report on this phenomenon). There is competition for status and power between people within the village. It amounts to each family striving to climb up the local hierarchical ladder of authority and dominance. Families of a lineage and/or neighbourhood may come together to form an alliance to protect themselves against powerful rivals. Families may come together because of affinal ties as reported for a village near Jodhpur by Bose and Malhotra (1964).

The significance of numbers in the village community has been sufficiently highlighted by Srinivas' (1959) concept of the dominant caste. He has observed that the ability to 'field' a number of able-bodied men is an important criterion for one's dominant position. Mandelbaum (1970) substantiates the status of a *jati* in its numerical strength in villages (see his description of alliances and factions). Instances where scores are settled in favour of a numerically-dominant caste have been cited by Srinivas (1959), Atal (1968) and others in their studies of villages in different parts of India. Studies conducted in the field of fertility in rural India (Wyon and Gordon 1971 and Mamdani 1972) have also reported the importance of numerical strength to a caste or clan, especially for faction fights. The latter two studies of the famous Khanna villages in Ludhiana district have reported on people's perception that bitter faction fights in villages are won by men, not contraceptives.

Mandelbaum (1970) has reported that factional quarrels are endemic to villages and that only a large united lineage or family can be confident of safeguarding status and interests. Fertility provides numerical strength and social status to a lineage or a *jati*. The primary interests augmented by fertility are located within the household and the family. We have seen earlier in this chapter the nature of economic aspirations parents harbour about their children. Here I wish to say that having several children, especially sons, is a sure protection for parents against denigrations and depredations. This does not mean that couples have chldren with the primary and explicit purpose of deriving political advantage. Similar observations have been made on other communities in India and elsewhere (Mamdani 1972 on Punjab; Caldwell 1982 on Africa; Cain 1977 on Bangladesh; Nag, Peet and White 1978 on Java and Nepal.)

Fertility is perceived as bringing status, prosperity and

numerical strength. Enhancement of parents' status in the household, their strength and standing in the wider society, their interaction with outsiders, and their ability to earn more and to help others, if need be, are some of the direct advantages parents experience through having children. With an increase in the status of a member of a household or family, the status of elders of the household, the family and relatives also increases. The larger the household, family and lineage, the greater the prestige of its senior members. Their sphere of authority widens as the lineage enlarges itself. More people approach them for help in matters such as labour exchange, borrowing money, and influencing government and other officials for expediting some pending matters in favour of those with fewer, and by implication less influential, members in the household.

Larger households enjoy a number of other advantages. They are likely to have more educated members holding salaried jobs and having contacts with government officials. The elders in these households frequently exercise their power through the younger members of their household and family. Many people approach them for their children's and grandchildren's marital alliances. People call on them to socialize. Since their network of relatives is wider than that of the others, more people interact with them. Thus, high fertility (birth of boys as well as of girls) is a politically beneficial venture both for parents and grandparents. A larger family means a larger gathering of kin and affines on ritual and ceremonial occasions, which enhances the status of the family. (See Caldwell 1982 and Shah and Desai 1988, for similar observations on Africa and India respectively. Lewis 1958 in his study of Rampur village near Delhi also reports that the assembly of a large number of relatives for a marriage party is an indication of one's power and influence.)

Being related to a large number of people and meeting them from time to time is a sign of a household's prestige. Kinship links with such a household are useful for all kinds of purposes, such as marital alliances for children and grandchildren, political alliances, capital accumulation, meeting economic and farming setbacks, security against unemployment, help in illness, and above all, sharing with insiders and denying to outsiders vital information and experiences of all kinds. The kinship and affinal connections are frequently invoked on occasions of rites of passage, such as birth, wedding and death.

Respect and honour in the community are important for precedence and dominance, which are earned by maintaining kinship and affinal and neighbourhood ties. Lorimer (1954) and Davis and Blake (1956) argue that families with several children may gain economic strength through political clout in local decision-making organizations. Caldwell (1982) raises an important question to understand the vital relevance of extended kinship ties: What do people want to do with their lives? Honour, esteem, affection, and pleasure are attained by spending on the extended family and the community.

A large network of relatives usually supports its members in adversity, such as morbidity, migration and unemployment. Srinivas (1978) observes that customary practices represent, among other things, people's social and psychological insurance in an extremely hostile world. Caldwell (1982: 35) further elaborates that political prestige is attained by cultivating the network of relatives and the cooperating group. Political success depends on the ability to tap more or better communal resources, increasing the number of people attending family ceremonies, and magnifying one's social importance. Kinship and other social relations are so dominant that a material transaction is usually a momentary episode in continuous social relations, observes Sahlins (1972: 185–6).

Besides the social and emotional advantages of having several children, affinal alliances are forged with members of other larger and socially-prestigious families to strengthen one's social standing. Parents with several children have numerous alliances in terms of their children's and grandchildren's affines. These usually stand by whenever a need arises.

> Vinji, an old Patel woman in her fifties, has seven children and 25 grandchildren (sons' and daughters' children). Five of her children were married into families in Mogra. Similarly, she has in Mogra a number of near and distant affines arising out of marriages of the 25 grandchildren. She also has many affinally-related people in the neighbouring villages. Vinji is thus related to numerous families in one way or another in and around the village.

In the village she belongs to the complex network of kin and affinal relatives and has direct access to a number of households. A fairly large number of people in the village, mostly consanguinous and affinal relatives, expressed concern and respect for her.

As most of the social and economic activities in the village are woven around the family, relatives and the community, a person with a large number of relatives is better placed than others. Having no children or having only one or two restricts one's sphere of interaction. There are only a few people to take care of such parents in adversity. Whatever be the occasional internal rifts in the family, its members stand united as a cohesive group when others pose a threat to its prestige and economic interests.

Baa, a Patel in his sixties, has five sons, one daughter and 27 grandchildren. On the other hand, his younger brother has only one son and two daughters. Whenever there are rifts between the two brothers' families, usually pertaining to farm produce or social obligations, Baa generally has an upper hand as all his sons (including those separated from his household) and grandsons stand by him. His younger brother cannot push matters forthrightly as he is aware that with fewer hands he cannot guard his property, fields and produce with the same efficiency and vigilance as Baa can. Even though people generally disapprove Baa's usual high-handedness, they rarely come out against him in public as his numerical strength is quite formidable. To antagonize Baa is to face the anger of his entire lot. People praise Baa's younger brother for his forbearance on social occasions, but they rarely fear him because his effective strength compared to that of Baa is insignificant.

Local dominance and precedence come more easily with a larger number of children. With more people's support, parents make their presence felt. Local dominance helps to sway people, even if the dominant group is unjust in its claims.

Pemji, a shepherd in his forties, has only two surviving daughters out of seven daughters and two sons born. His elder brother, on the other hand, has three sons and two daughters. Due to his and his wife's illness, Pemji was heavily indebted. Consequently he wished to sell a part of his land to repay some of his debts. But his elder brother has been obstructing all his moves for nearly a decade. The land is in Pemji's deceased father's name. For any land deal, both brothers have to come together. Pemji cannot convince his brother who knows that the land will belong to him and his sons one day. If Pemji had a few sons, he would not have been indebted nor felt the need to dispose of the land.

Pemji's case shows the plight of a sonless household. It is not enough to have a child to absolve parents of the curse of barrenness. In the absence of a son, parents may lose effective control over their own property.

The problems faced by a lone person or by parents with only one son are reflected in the adge: '*ēkaliya ree hēday charē*' (literally, the cattle of a lone person always graze on the periphery). In other words, it is easy to brush aside a lone person. This is a metaphorical explanation of the weakness of those having fewer children.

Movni, a 25-year-old Jat woman, explained to me the importance of high fertility and the need for a minimum of two sons by asking: 'Can a single piece of wood burn if put in the hearth? Only two, rather three or four of them put together burn well.' She also explained: 'However much there are quarrels among household and family members, they stand as a united front against any outsider. Outsiders generally think twice before attacking or harming any member of a large family, while a lone person may be attacked any time. For people going to work in the fields the company and security provided by family members are essential.'

Fertility leading to the birth of several sons is as crucial as fire in a hearth in a house. By implication, one can live better only with a few sons.

Hari, a young mother in her twenties, has two young daughters and a three-year-old son. She lives in a complex household comprising herself, her husband, three children and her mother-in-law. The husband works as a tractor driver and is away most of the time. The work on the family's farm is done mostly by Hari and her mother-in-law. Puni is Hari's neighbour and has three sons and two daughters, all married. One son looks after the land, while her husband and two other sons manage a grocery shop in Jodhpur city. Puni takes pride in the fact that her large family owns not only land but also a shop. On one occasion, Hari's cattle strayed into Puni's land. A scuffle broke out between the two and Puni was roughed up. Puni retorted with innuendoes against Hari's husband and ridiculed the two women for having to manage the family's land. The absence of men to work on her land was a degrading fact in Hari's life. But she claimed that she would one day be a mother of 12 sons and be in a position to settle scores.

Even though Hari is physically stronger than Puni, the fact that the latter has more children confers a superior status on her. But for such a drawback the older and weaker Puni would never have dared challenge Hari in the field. Later Hari was widely criticized for her disrespect towards the elderly Puni.

The above cases illustrate that larger families are generally associated with prosperity, politicial strength and influence. We have already seen that a family's influence increases not only with the birth of several sons but also with that of daughters. Although a daughter leaves her natal home upon marriage, her affinal alliance helps her natal household to enlarge the network of relatives. A daughter helps enhance her natal household's social position through affinal alliances with other politically- and economically-influential households. The influence of fathers and brothers increases with the enlargement of the network of relatives in the village, the *chautāḷo*, and occasionally, even outside it. The religious and emotional value of daughters is well-known (discussed separately), but their social and political value is rarely highlighted in fertility studies. For instance, studies conducted by Wyon and Gordon (1971), Mamdani (1972) and Mandelbaum (1974) emphasize the political significance of sons in India but pay little attention to the value of daughters.

This should not, however, mean that couples in Mogra go on producing as many children as their fecundity permits. We have already seen in this and the previous chapter that household formation and fertility are mediated by convention. We shall see more of this pertaining to fertility control in Chapters 6 and 7.

### *Cosmology*

The prevalent fertility behaviour has an associated set of beliefs. Children have vital social and religious significance. Not only sons but daughters also enjoy a religious value in all caste groups. It is believed that one earns *punna* by giving away a daughter in marriage. A common saying is: 'The courtyard of a house should not remain virgin.' Its implication is that the marriage of at least one daughter must be performed in the courtyard. Couples without a daughter usually arrange for the wedding ritual and related expenses of an agnatic kin's daughter in their courtyard to earn *punna*. Shah (1973: 17) refers to the deeply ingrained belief about the marriage of a daughter bringing religious merit in Gujarat. Giving gifts to daughters by parents and to sisters by brothers on various occasions throughout their lives is believed to bring not only social honour but also *punna*. If there are several brothers, they share their obligation toward sisters.

The ritual importance of a son is demonstrated uniformly in all castes, although there are variations pertaining to details in rituals. It is strongly belieived that sons are important to continue the family name by maintaining the patriline. The absence of a son is compensated by the practice of adoption and also of *ghar jamāi* (among some castes). Sons bring *moksha* (liberation from the cycle of birth and rebirth; ultimate salvation) to deceased parents. Sons light the funeral pyre, take their parents' ashes to the holy Ganga for *moksha* (locally called *gati*; actually short form of *sadgati*). Harijans too practise this but not as elaborately as the other castes. Sons organize mortuary feasts upon their old parents' death. Feeding people on such an occasion brings religious merit both to the deceased and to the host of the mortuary feast, besides enhancing the status of the household.

If parents have a large number of children they consider themselves to be fortunate. Fecundity is god's gift. If it was not so there would have been no sterility, they argue. Sterility is considered a curse. It leads to termination of life. Fertility is thus a divine blessing. It brings a sense of completeness and ful-fillment to a couple, a purpose and relevance to life. It leads to prosperity and well-being in the present and the other world. It is through one's children that one's name and memory get perpetuated. The customary practice of reading out genealogical records of one's lineage and clan ancestors upon every new entry in one's genealogist's register is zealously practised. The records are a valued possession and are an important component of one's cherished treasure kept in the custody of genealogists.[4]

---

[4] Members of the caste of genealogists, called Rav or Bhat, live in other villages in the region and visit their patrons in Mogra for the purpose of updating the records in their registers. They visit Mogra once or twice a year. See Shah and Shroff (1958) for an account of such a caste in adjoining Gujarat state.

A house full of children in compared to a flowering tree and is a source of parents' pride. Children symbolize prosperity and happiness. It is rare to find a household without children. Such a household is considered unfortunate and unbearably desolate, one that pounces upon one like a glutton (*khāli ghar khāvanē dauḍe*). Not having children implies that a person is unable to continue one's patriline which is clearly a disrespect to one's ancestors. By producing children, especially sons, one repays one's ancestral debt.

An open door signifies a happy household, full of people. There are, however, customary practices (adoption and *ghar jamāi*) that enable an individual to overcome the problems associated with not having a son. Discharge of kinship and ritual obligations needs a large number of children. The need for sons in Hindu society is well known. The son in all caste groups has a number of functions to perform in relation to his parents, siblings and sister's children. A major responsibility of children towards parents is to take the ashes of the deceased parents to the Ganga. It also involves arranging the mortuary feast discussed in Chapter 1. A son's other responsibilities after parents' death are to bring up the younger siblings, get them married and, as already mentioned, in case of sisters, to arrange for obligatory gifts on various occasions throughout their lives. The obligations toward sisters can be shared if there are several brothers. The total number of gifts received by a sister is also large if she has more than one brother, which enhance her standing in the conjugal home.

The ritual and symbolic significance of children to parents is found in their status enhancement through birth itself. Right from the time of birth, the child begins to add to the parents' and the household's status. The domestic, economic, political and ritual spheres are symbolically interlinked in the cosmology that reinforces the positive value of fertility.

CHAPTER 4

# *Culture and Social Organization of Childbirth*

Childbirth in Mogra is not burden on the husband-wife couple alone, but a responsibility of the entire household. It is organized socially, in sharp contrast to modern society. The identity of the couple is subordinated to that of the household when the network of mutual help and sharing is mobilized for the purpose of organizing childbirth. In other words, the entire household is a unit in the network of reciprocity. It is therefore fully adept at handling childbirth without suspending other matters and schedules.

Although the mother suffers the physical pain of childbirth, her suffering is substantially contained because relatives, neighbours and the wider community pool their resources. These resources consist essentially of mutual help and sharing provided by people through their physical presence, and willingness to help the couple in any work at any time. The community resources are the various local beliefs and practices which people have been employing for a long time to ensure successful childbirth.

The pregnant woman's significance for the household, the family and the community is expressed in several ways. The various institutionalized practices during pregnancy and childbirth indicate the high value society places on procreation.

For a woman pregnancy and childbirth, especially the first child's birth and/or a son's birth, leads to her status graduation and is accompanied by important rites of passage (see Van Gennep 1960 on how thresholds symbolize the beginning of new statuses).

The cosmology that routinizes pregnancy and contains the

intensity of labour pain serves several purposes. It keeps anxiety and hysteria under control. The informal networks and inexpensive infrastructure for child delivery prevent it from being an exhorbitant proposition. The intimate and active participation of the household and other relatives reinforces the woman's emotional and moral make-up. The rituals associated with childbirth periodically convert the obligatory into the desirable. These are what Bernstein (1977: 55) calls, 'consensual rituals' inasmuch as they function to bind together community members and transmit and reinforce society's central value system. Rituals have highly condensed and predictable messages, and have extra verbal or indirect meanings. They are a form of 'restricted code'. They evoke organization of sentiments and revivify the social order within the individual (see Giddens' 1984 account of actors' 'knowledgeability' to go on in society, and the mutual monitoring of behaviour). Rituals accord public acclaim to a new mother for her favour to the household. Both the infant and the new mother are assigned a high value during birth-associated rituals.

Child delivery and the ensuing confinement are called *jāpa*, literally, a combination of two words, *jaa*, meaning birth, and *paa*, meaning to receive. A new mother is said to be in a state of *jāpa* and thus called a *jāpaiti*. The term childbirth, as used here, means *jāpa*. A *jāpāiti* not only gives by way of childbirth but receives as well. Her gains are both material and symbolic. Her child is her highest reward. In addition, she receives extraordinary care and attention. The *huāvaḍ*, i.e., herbal sweets prepared in ghee, are culturally valued as among the best of foods. It is a special reward for the *jāpāiti*, as it is meant specially for her, and is also served to her in bed. She is treated with special care both in terms of food and rest. The younger woman who generally consumes stale and left-over food, finds the *huāvaḍ* an exciting change after child delivery. A *jāpāiti* is on complete bed rest, otherwise seldom permitted. She is fully relieved of arduous chores. Both valued food and rest are rare luxury for a woman, but are available to a new mother. She also receives gifts from various relatives and friends. On attaining motherhood, her status graduates in the household and the community.

It may be clarified that the experience of *jāpa* and *huāvaḍ* is not uniform for all castes in Mogra. Many poor people cannot afford these to the same extent as the rich. For instance, Harijan women rarely have access to rich *huāvaḍ* prepared in ghee like upper caste women. Their *huāvaḍ* is usually prepared in oil, proscribed for other *jāpāitis*. Their post-partum rest is also shorter. Of course, given their resources, *jāpa* and *huāvaḍ* are a luxury for Harijan women too.

*Huāvaḍ* holds a special value in the scale of food specialities in village life. Most women relish it. They look forward to an opportunity to have it. It is a form of sweets, generally called *lādu*, prepared in ghee with a variety of herbs. It is believed to have special medicinal value for a *jāpāiti*. Women eat it only during physical crisis, say childbirth. On other occasions an old woman with ailments such as knee-pain, backache and arthritis can have *lādu*. As opportunities to have them are few, they are greatly desired. It is common for a woman to ask another; 'When are you going to have *lādu*?' and 'When would you sleep?' Meaning when is the baby due?

### *Attitudes Towards Pregnancy*

Pregnancy in Mogra is considered a normal and desirable condition for a young woman. Laderman observes the same for rural Malaysia, where pregnancy 'requires few changes in behaviour (and) is expected to proceed on a largely uneventful course to its ultimate conclusion' (1983: 119). For most of the gestation period a pregnant woman is hardly given any major concession in the physical work expected of her. Only during the last trimester, is she dissuaded from lifting heavy loads, of say, 15 to 20 kg. However, she may carry a pitcher of water, after it is placed on her head by someone else. She is encouraged to grind grains with a hand mill (*ghatti*), which is believed to prepare her for smooth delivery. It is commonly believed that regular physical activity facilitates labour and makes child delivery less painful.

The pregnant woman's diet remains by and large the same as that of other women, though the amount of intake is expected to increase. The prevailing justification is: 'The one inside also needs food.' Certain food cravings are usually associated with pregnancy. This qualifies a woman to get most of her cravings fulfilled, which is denied a non-pregnant woman. In the culture of austerity characterizing this village society, a woman's normal diet consists of certain staple items. But a pregnant woman is exempted from this rule. In normal times little concern is shown for a woman's food preferences. During pregnancy, however, the concern for her palate is an indication of the importance accorded to her physiological state. To satisfy a pregnant woman's food cravings is to earn *punna*, as the food is consumed not only by the woman but also by the growing foetus. Relatives, friends and neighbours make a conscious attempt to satisfy her cravings, as this earns them not only *punna* but, more visibly, social appreciation as well. The belief supports the view that a foetus also has the status of a normal living being. The concern a pregnant woman enjoys is extended indirectly to her foetus as well. Unattended food cravings of the foetus are believed to carry over to its infancy, so much so that it is considered possible to distinguish whether an infant was satiated or not when it was in the womb. One supposedly distinguishing feature is the infant's ability to control the frequent dribbling of saliva from its mouth. A baby with regular dribbling of saliva is considered as one whose cravings were not fulfilled during its embryonic stage. Women often say of such a baby: 'What craving did your mother not express (which left you uncontented)?'

Attending to a pregnant woman's food cravings is institutionalized by the ritual of *hād purāṇo*, literally, to attend to the pregnant woman's taste. This includes a sumptuous treat given by close relatives, neighbours and friends in turn. In addition, some sweets and clothes are also gifted by close relatives, particularly the mother-in-law, during the seventh month of the first pregnancy. These practices wane in their intensity and observance at subsequent pregnancies. Many pregnant women pick up the habit of chewing pieces of *mate* (fuller's earth, a pale coloured hard clay available at grocery shops). Though this habit is not quite approved, it is not discouraged firmly either. However, if it is not terminated soon after child delivery, it is strongly disapproved.

The nature of food cravings is believed to offer important clues to the sex of the prospective baby. Usually, they are categorized as sweet and sour. The former connotes the birth of a son, while the latter that of a daugher, although the outcome does not necessarily follow the belief.

Much of the anxiety associated with pregnancy among urban middle class women does not exist among women in Mogra. As mentioned in Chapter 3, the knowledge about childbearing is derived much early in life through various customs and observations in the household and the neighbourhood. For instance, it is common for children to see domestic animals like cows, buffaloes, sheep and goats giving birth. Children around 10 years of age, particularly girls, often assist their parents in attending to cattle that are about to calve in a day or two. Children growing up with such experiences attain some basic understanding of biological reproduction. (See Erikson 1950 for a discussion of how children emulate adult roles, and how all people start as children.) Similarly, the girls of the household assist a *dai* (lower caste midwife) and other birth attendants waiting upon a labouring woman. If not very young (below 10 years), girls are permitted to remain in the vicinity of the labouring woman. Such an exposure provides first-hand knowledge of the process of child delivery. Adolescent girls observe such events in the case of their mothers, aunts, sisters and brother's wives even before they themselves reach the stage of delivering children.

The common image of a labouring woman in Mogra is one who endures her agony silently. The not-yet-mothers appropriate this image much early in life. Young girls witness child deliveries and overhear adult women discussing pregnancies and child deliveries occurring in their neighbourhood. A woman facing prolonged labour pain knows what is expected of her and of those attending on her. Her intimate understanding of the situation helps keep anxiety and hysteria at bay. Child delivery is handled with a matter-of-course attitude, and this indeed is the cultural ideal.

As already noted in Chapter 3, young women seldom discuss their conception and pregnancy with elders. Also, teenaged married women seldom respond to queries about their pregnancy unless they are fully assured that their responses will not be disclosed. Such issues are talked about only with a few intimate friends or relatives. Senior women draw necessary information about the pregnancy of young women, especially about the first pregnancy, through the latter's close friends. Even evasion of questions put to a young woman about her pregnancy is a part of her modesty.

> When I asked pregnant Sukhi about the probable month when her first child was due, she diverted the subject by asking me to have food. When prodded she said evasively: 'It will happen on its own. I don't know. Please don't ask me such embarrassing questions.'

### *Child Delivery Practices*

Actual child delivery is exclusively a women's affair. Care is taken to see that men do not participate either by way of knowing or by being present near the labouring woman. Child delivery is usually conducted by some elderly women relatives or neighbours who have the knowledge and prior experience of handling births. A *dai* is also called. The attendants and the *dai* together manage the delivery. The *dai* is rarely considered to be such an expert that her every advice has to be followed. Except in difficult cases, such as when the mother's life is in danger, a professionally-trained nurse is rarely summoned. There has been only one occasion in the past few decades in Mogra when a doctor was summoned to conduct a child delivery. Modern medicine is not quickly resorted to. 'Wait and see' is the people's attitude. People resort to modern medicine only when a woman's life is threatened and the local birth attendants fail to handle the complications. Since child delivery is almost always considered to be normal, and rarely to be dangerous, the waiting period is usually prolonged.

> Rambha, a young Raika woman, was brought to Mogra from her natal village after having labour pains for a few days without delivery. Her parents-in-law in Mogra were in a quandary. Several others got to know about the case soon. On the advice of a few influential educated persons she was taken to a hospital in Jodhpur city. She delivered a baby soon after reaching the hospital. Upon getting to know about the normal delivery, her relatives reiterated that it was merely a matter of time and the panic was unnecessary.

A *dai* is called usually for the first two deliveries. Later, she is invited only if the household cannot handle it with its own human and material resources. Although a trained nurse attached to the dispensary in Mogra lives in the village, a *dai* is preferred to her for several reasons. A *dai* is adept in the local tradition of conducting child deliveries which is more acceptable to people. Unlike the professional nurse she is always available and will not say 'no' even when sent for at odd hours. Her services are not even half as expensive as the nurse's, and the same is true of her medicines. In addition, a *dai* offers several additional services not performed by the nurse, such as cleaning the effluvia and placenta, performing various rituals related to burying the placenta, cleaning the place and purifying it with dung paste, bathing the baby, sponging the mother, making her bed, washing her clothes and giving post-natal massage. Above all, a *dai* accepts payment in both cash and kind. In kind she is given meals, foodgrains, old garments, a piece of new cloth, and a ball of herbal sweets prepared for the parturient mother. Payment in instalments dispersed over long periods of time seems more reasonable to the people than a one-time payment of cash to the nurse for a shorter visit. People say that the nurse is more bothered about her fees, and has little consideration for a client with limited resources. A *dai*, on the other hand, accepts though not always ungrudgingly, whatever little is paid by those with meagre resources.

As child delivery is expected to follow a normal course for all women, no fear or anxiety associated with it is blown out of proportion. In the same vein, spending money on child delivery is considered improper. Accordingly, the nurse is summoned only when the relatives and the *dai* have exhausted all their methods. Even when a nurse is brought in at such a moment she is asked to wait for a few minutes and is prevented from giving any medicine or an injection, to avoid payment.

> Ansi was labouring for her second child and the nurse had to be summoned because of certain complications. She was asked to wait for about 15 minutes, and prevented from administering any medicine. She was permitted only to examine Ansi's abdomen. After some time when Ansi delivered a boy, her mother-in-law asked the nurse to quit. She was not paid anything for her midnight visit. The reason given by Ansi's parents-in-law was that she had given no medicine and a mere visit did not entitle her to any payment.

Usually, the senior female relatives conducting child delivery are never paid anything for the work, but they are a part of the broader network of gift exchange by virtue ofbeing relatives or neighbours.

The same reasoning for non-payment is applied to the nurse as well, even if the nurse is hardly a part of the gift exchange network.

> Two years after Ansi had her second baby she was due for childbirth and had the same complications during labour. All her attendants felt the need to call the nurse. Her *jēthani* went to summon her. The nurse first made sure that this time she did not wait beside Ansi till she was delivered of her baby. She made it clear that she would begin her medication soon after examining Ansi and claim a fee. It was only on this condition that she agreed to move out of her house.'

Both the people and the nurse are not used to each other's code of conduct. Each is critical of the other's conduct. Gradually, the people are adapting to the nurse's demands, albeit after a great deal of procrastination and resistance. She is also learning to deal with village ways.

> The nurse related her experiences in Mogra: 'I overcharge for the medicine because these people pay only for medicine and never for services. I put the two together and show it as the cost of medicine. They prefer to bargain even after this, and usually pay much less than asked for. And they pay in instalments. They never pay in one go.'
>
> Roopi Raika beed for three days before delivering a feeble baby. The female relatives attending on her were all afraid she would die, but they did not summon a nurse or a doctor because a certain hope lingered on, that everything would be normal. Also, they thought that professional help would be beyond the reach of the poor household. However, with a normal delivery their hopes were not belied.
>
> Umaji's wife was in bed for 23 days with an enormous swelling all over her body that disabled movement. In the last few days of her ailment, the *dai* and a *Grām-Sēwak* (village-level worker) warned the household elders that there was urgent need of a doctor, because to them the case was rather serious. Even the nurse who had conducted her previous child delivery had warned the household that the next child delivery would endanger her life. Despite these warnings, the decision to take her to hospital was made too late. Before she could reach the city hospital she succumbed. Later people realized how serious and dangerous such a swelling could be during pregnancy. Her mother-in-law later lamented, 'She used to have this kind of swelling during every pregnancy. Even this time I thought it was the same, and that she would be normal once she delivered the baby.' Umaji could not find another wife for himself even till two years later.

Besides the above there were two other cases of maternal mortality fresh in people's memory. Both the young women had come to their natal homes in Mogra for their first confinements. Four other cases of maternal mortality were reported (discussed in Chapter 5). These cases have, however, not brought much change in people's outlook towards child delivery.

Child delivery is rarely feared as a major uncertainty. After the first two child deliveries, several women are confident of handling it easily, and all alone if the occasion arises.

> Keli, a Harijan woman, gave birth to eight children, four of whom survived. She said: 'When my first child was to be born, a *dai*, who was also my relative, was sent for. After some time, the *dai* felt that the case was too complicated for her. She suggested that the nurse be called. The nurse gave me two injections and I had a stillbirth. After that, my people never called the nurse. The remaining seven deliveries took place with the help of the *dai* and without any complications. The *dai* was summoned only as a precaution.' Keli explained with a proverb: 'Obviously infants don't drop from one's ear (*kaun mūn nee khirē*).' This proverb is commonly used to indicate that even though child delivery is not an uphill task, it is no child's play either.
>
> Phooli, a Patel woman, came with her newly-born baby in her arms from the field a kilometre away. When I asked why she did not come home when the labour pains began, she said: 'The pain was bearable and irregular. So I thought the delivery was a few hours away. I continued to chop *bajri* stalks. Suddenly the pains shot up. I could hardly move to a smoother ground. As I squatted, the baby was born. I cut the umbilical cord with a sickle, buried the effluvia there itself, tore a piee of my *orno* (half-saree) and wrapped the baby in it, and set out for home with the baby. She is my fifth child, but the first I had all alone. I felt a strange courage in me to face it all by myself. God was kind enough to make it so smooth for me.'
>
> On being asked whether she didn't lose heart, Phooli said: 'We are much better off. The Jogis and Nats (the nomadic castes) have all their child deliveries outside their homes while they are wandering. Their women rarely get any rest, nor do they get proper *huavaḍ* and yet they are strong and sturdy.'
>
> Gajari, another Patel woman, also delivered her second baby on her way home from the field.

By the third and subsequent child deliveries the matter-of-course attitude towards childbirth becomes more marked as is evident from some of the above cases. By repeated births, mothers acquire sufficient knowledge and courage to deliver babies all alone at home and even in the fields.

Through the custom of the woman's first confinement in the natal, and the subsequent ones in the conjugal house, the two households share the expenses, in addition to providing physical, social and moral support to the expectant woman. For the first confinement, called *paṇi pāvaṇo* or *jāpa mātē lāvṇo* (literally, to serve water, or to bring the girl for confinement) she is brought to her natal home during the last trimester of pregnancy. The first delivery in the natal home is believed to be more congenial for the young pregnant woman. It requires greater emotional care, always available in the natal home. In the conjugal home, on the other hand, a young wife has to observe *gungto* and cannot communicate directly with the elders, which is a serious inconvenience to her. In the natal home, she can be more frank, which is believed to be a prerequisite for successful childbirth. In addition, it is socially and religiously meritorious for the natal kin to help a daughter deliver her first child. All the expenses of conducting the first childbirth and *huāvaḍ* are borne by the natal kin. Gifts for the infant, the new mother and her conjugal relatives are additional customary obligations. This is the responsibility of a woman's parents, and in their absence, of her brothers. Only an orphaned woman, with no one in the parental home, has to deliver her first child in her conjugal home. Such cases are rare. In Mogra only one woman had such an experience.

The first childbirth provides deeper moorings to the young mother in her conjugal household, and prepares her for the second childbirth there. In this case, all expenses for childbirth and a part of *huāvaḍ* have to be borne by the conjugal household. A few weeks after the second child's birth the natal relatives bring her a variant of *huāvaḍ* called *paḍodi*. The institution is called *lādu lāṇa*, literaly, to bring sweet balls. The pot containing *paḍodi* is opened before a gathering of relatives and others for display and comment. On the whole, this institution reduces the expenditure on *huāvaḍ* for the conjugal household. It is only in the third and subsequent childbirths that the conjugal household bears the entire expenditure. If an assessment of expenses is made for the first three childbirths of a woman, it will be found that her natal and conjugal households have contributed almost equally. By this time the woman has a considerable say in her conjugal household. She is no longer a girl but a fullfledged woman and mother.

A proper recognition of membership in the conjugal household comes to a woman only through birth of children and their survival. Her natal kin actively participate in enabling her to achieve that status by conducting her first child delivery. In case the first infant dies before the new mother reaches her conjugal home after confinement, the second confinement also takes place in the natal home. Thus, her total acceptance in the conjugal household becomes possible only on being the mother of a suriving child. Papanek (1973) observes that a woman's personal worth is related to her fertility performance and she attains status by being the mother of a number of children, especially sons. Srinivas and Ramaswamy (1977) are of the view that the status of a newly-married woman in her conjugal household is primarily one of a bearer of children. Patel observes: 'Her primary role at this stage is of wife-mother, and her success in this role is directly reflected in the number of living children she has (1982: 370).'

The larger network of relatives participate symbolically in the event of childbirth. The parturient mother becomes ritually impure. This extends temporarily to all other members of the household. Their temporary ritual impurity is the state of *hutak* (a derivation from Sanskrit *sutaka*, strongly associated with birth impurity). Even when the first childbirth takes place in the woman's natal house, *hutak* is believed to spread not only to members of that household but also to those of her conjugal household. The latter formally observe ritual impurity. There are prohibitions against contact and against accepting water and food from those in a state of *hutak*. Others are vulnerable to pollution by their contact. The participation of kin and affines in various ways gives the pregnant and the parturient woman a feeling of security and importance. She is not left to fend for herself.

### *Cosmology of Childbirth and the Social Structure*

The manner in which child delivery is conducted in Mogra prevents it from being an experience of travail and trauma. The attendants take every care to comfort, support and reassure the labouring woman. Their indigenous skills of child delivery and the emotional framework they provide boost the morale of the labouring woman whose strength intermittently flags. She rarely writhes in pain all by herself.[1] She is the centre of attention for all those present beside her in the privacy of the room. They all in volve themselves intensively with her. Their frisky movements, pauses, sounds, talk and facial expressions are in accordance with the woman's rhythm of pain, and give her much-needed strength and encouragement. Their serious participation in the process indicates that the child is desired by them collectively and that the mother is performing a heroic personal as well as social ordeal. The people around provide mechanisms that effectively prevent the labouring woman from turning hysterical or even losing her calm. The warmth of collective participation and emotional care is in sharp contrast to that experienced by labouring women in British hospitals which affects them adversely (Kitzinger 1982, Stephens 1986). Stephens argues that an absolute non-recognition of the emotional framework, or elimination of the woman's effort at child delivery (encapsulated within the medical jurisdiction), makes childbirth inadequate and robs the mother of a sense of achievement by minimizing her participation.

As the entire household is geared up around the labouring mother, she feels immensely important. During labour, any female member of her household or the neighbourhood can assist in the numerous tasks related to childbirth. During the crisis period of labour, the usual allocation of roles in the household based on seniority and kinship is relaxed liberally. Every woman of the household does her best to carry out whatever task is required for successful childbirth, irrespective of her status vis-a-vis the labouring woman and the nature of the task. This applies to the

---

[1] Stephens in her paper, 'The Childbirth Industry: A Woman's View' (1986) gives spine-chilling examples of Indian female gynaecologists and obstreticians often humiliating and insulting labouring women who have submitted to their professional supremacy at the cost of their own psychological well-being. Kitzinger (1982) describes the feeling of alienation from their bodies and the deprivation of autonomy that women in labour experience in British hospitals.

natal, as well as the conjugal, household. Senior women usually do jobs which are not expected of them during normal times, especially in relation to junior members, including daughters-in-law. A *jēthaṇi*, *naṇand* (husband's sister) and even mother-in-law may hold a labouring woman's legs and give her a wash and massage. She can relax her *gūngto* before her mother-in-law or any other older conjugal woman. More often than not, she begins to talk directly to her mother-in-law during her second child delivery. Usually this serves as the ice-breaking point from when the daughter-in-law may begin to talk to her mother-in-law. The inversion is not considred a breach but the norm itself. Respect for older women is resumed by observing *gūngto* after childbirth. Many younger mothers with the experience of two or three child deliveries again refrain from talking to their mothers-in-law as a mark of respect.

A woman's pain is not just biological. Indeed there is nothing universal and objective about bodily sensations which convey accurately the extent of discomfort in pain. The experience of pain is highly conditioned by the mediation of cultural and social practices. Pain is both a fact and a value. Pain as a fact acquires different values in different cultures.[2] Pain is understood, experienced and responded to customarily. The socially-defined perception of pain and its appropriation at the subjective level plays a crucial role in understanding and controlling it or in relenting under it. For instance, in an urban middle class context, a small cut or bruise might be considered a serious matter, with an associated fear of tetanus needing quick medical attention such as a bandage, ointment or an injection. In contrast, such cuts and bruises are overlooked as matter of course in Mogra. A little sand on a cut is all that the remedy consists of. A similar response to pain in child delivery is conditioned partly by the strong influcence of cultural training, a matter-of-course perception, and its frequent occurrence (at home) in a society with high fertility. People are accustomed to experiencing and handling child delivery without fear, panic and uncertainty. Unlike in modern society,

[2] Sontag (1979: 44) illustrates how discases like tuberculosis and cancer are positively metaphored and the sick are appreciated for possessing certain qualities.

pregnancy and child delivery are not a major cause for anxiety, expenditure, and dependence on medical expertise (see Greer 1984, for a contrast between the urban west and rural east in this regard).

For the woman in Mogra, labour pain is an inevitable aspect of the desirable and obligatory part of her life cycle. It is seen as a means to a prospective end. Pain during childbirth is considered a natural burden and a necessary evil that has to be endured. Childbirth might be physically painful but the prestige and high social value attached to motherhood glorifies the experience. Childbirth is a prelude to enhanced status and not to physical degeneration. Women are aware that a more favourable and comfortable situation awaits them as soon as they are through with labour. The pleasantness associated with the outcome neutralizes the intensity of pain.

A labouring woman's control over her situation is facilitated by the prevailing cosmology. Certain practices in a woman's everyday life embody the cosmology of suffering that enables her to tide over labour pains. Illich rightly points out: 'In one way or another all cultures teach suffering as an art enabling one to deal in . . . the kind of physical pain that cannot be avoided' (1975: 94). A strong belief in Mogra eases the difficulty of child delivery. A woman's fearless and heroic control over herself during child delivery is explained in terms of certain desirable humane personality attributes. It is believed that good, affectionate, loving, selfless, saintly and simple souls have easy child deliveries. Those women who care for other's needs and comforts experience painless child delivery. Well-meaning women with sincere thoughts and deeds never face any problems during labour. On the other hand, wicked, cunning, selfish, miserly, non-loving, greedy, quarrelsome and mean women are sure to suffer difficulties and complications.

Several magical beliefs and rituals are practised for successful child delivery. For instance, when a daughter-in-law proceeds to her natal home for her first confinement, a *mauḷi* (a sacred and protective thread believed to bring well-being) is tied on her right wrist. Her mother-in-law performs the ritual of *khoḷ bharāvaṇo* (literally, to fill the lap). She places some sweets, a coconut and some money in the pregnant daughter-in-law's *pallo* (one end of the saree) spread across her lap. The latter carries the sweets and other items to her natal home. After placing them at the shrine of household deities, they are distributed among children (see Douglas 1960: 71–2 for a discussion on people's perception of the efficacy of magical beliefs and rituals).

Pregnant women are encouraged to give alms and be kind to others so as to avoid complications during child delivery. Even during labour they are advised to take vows and declare that upon successful delivery they would give as alms some amount of grains to birds, Saads and Brahmins, and some fodder to cattle. Taking such vows is believed to be an aid in child delivery.[3] This observation is similar to Laderman's (1983: 51) exposition of the Malay belief that complications during labour are experienced by women who stray from their feminine role—such as being subordinate to the husband in thought and deed during the period of pregnancy. The belief in Mogra may be partly contrasted with that in Malaysia. In Mogra, women's role relates to the larger society and not simply to their husbands. Women are expected to be better human beings and not simply better wives. The belief is so deeply internalized that labouring women consciously suppress their anguish to avoid being labelled as bad. They set an example of courage and fortitude. Even summoning any outside help is avoided as long as possible. Calling a *dai* is considered the first signal of difficulty, while calling a nurse is a strong indication that the woman is not noble. After a few childbirths many women prefer to deliver their babies without a *dai*'s or nurse's help, to demonstrate that child delivery is not difficult. This practice is quite common and younger women emulate it in an attempt to be proximate to the ideal image.

Even when child delivery is not so easy, women deliberately project a contrary impression. To justify their summoning a *dai* or a nurse, some women blame their mother's anxiety to give an impression that the delivery is normal.

Jhammu told me: 'My body was cold and sweating and she (her

---

[3] As mentioned in the previous chapter, giving alms is believed to be an indication of one's religiosity. In the same vein, making a declaration to give alms is seen as a religious act. Invoking assistance from these sources during disease and difficulty is reported elsewhere (Srinivas 1952: Dube 1955).

mother) thought it was beyond me. I did not let the *dai* massage and press my abdomen. In fact, I delivered in no time after the *dai* arrived. My mother gets very restive. After all, mother's love is such'.

Self-control in the labouring woman during child delivery is constantly encouraged through the prevailing norms. A woman delivering a child while working in the fields is applauded and praised as a simple soul. The confidence and self-reliance perpetuates the belief that pregnancy and child delivery are a matter of routine in a woman's life.

Groaning and screaming during labour are disapproved. If a woman screams, she is severely criticized and immediately silenced by her attendants. Later, she has to face several uncomfortable queries which indirectly cast doubts on her positive attributes. On the while, labour pains are to be endured courageously with the hope to attaining successful motherhood and associated social status. Childbirth immediately accords new positions and roles to the new mother, father and other relatives. The infant is socially placed in the family as well as the larger community. Thus, when a woman attains motherhood, and her husband fatherhood, other relatives emerge as uncles, aunts and so on.

Another common belief is that child delivery becomes complicated and more painful as more and more people, especially men, get to learn of a woman labouring. A labouring woman's screams impede the process. It is believed that fewer the men knowing about a woman in labour the easier it is to deliver a baby. Louder groans are immediately stifled and the woman is reminded that if any man comes to know labour would be prolonged and painful. Even younger children around might come to know of the labour, it is feared. It may become difficult to restrain them from approaching the labouring woman. She is pacified and tenderly treated, but not allowed to groan and scream.

The openings of grain storages are loosened and the woman's hair is untied to symbolically accelerate labour. This practice has also been reported from a north Indian village by Jeffery *et al.* (1984). (See Douglas 1960: 58–72 for an elaboration of this point.) The labouring woman is asked to pray along with others around to Ve Mata, the deity of birth. Ve Mata is the wife of Brahma, the creator of the world. Her blessings help fruitful child delivery. She is believed to be the giver of life and the mother of all. She is solicited several times while the woman is in labour. She is importuned to come to the woman's rescue. A *chājḍo* (grain chaffing implement made of straw) containing grain and *guḍ* (jaggery) is paced beside the woman's head as an offering to Ve Mata. It is a way of symbolically welcoming her spirit. The practice of praying during labour among the Malay has similar functions. Laderman observes: 'Concentration on prayer rather than pain may lead a woman away from anxieties that can interfere with uterine functions. If incipient hysteria is cut off in its beginnings, and a satisfactory alternative substituted, it may be beneficial for the outcome of labour' (1983: 166).

Reversal of symbols take place during child delivery. The labouring woman is encouraged to repeat the names of her husband's parents and ancestors—an act disapproved in normal times. The insistence by elderly attendants on repeating these names is quite awkward for her and takes her mind off physical pain. She rarely questions the basic assumptions of cultural values, norms and knowledge. Instead, she accepts advice and directions sincerely, a trait also reported from Malaysia by Laderman (1983). The women around pray to the gods for her because it is assumed that the atmosphere at such a time is infested by evil spirits and demons who might prove harmful. They are prevented by invoking the divine to ward off possible danger. Prayers are offered to invoke the family and local deities to relieve the labouring woman by successful and speedy child delivery.

Mogra's cultural beliefs and practices consist of a framework of comfort and care which makes child delivery a simple and fearless affair. The pain and anxiety of child delivery are thus effectively dealt with. The pain is overcome substantially and sublimated symbolically as contrasted with child delivery experiences in a modern hospital (Kitzinger 1982; Greer 1984; Stephens 1986).

### *Material Resources for Child delivery*

Child delivery in Mogra requires very few material resources, compared to the paraphernalia in a maternity hospital. There is no elaborate preparation in terms of space, bedding, clothing and equipment. Prior appointment with a doctor is, of course, ruled out. The local *dai*, and expert women relatives, are already aware of the pregnancy. Usually they arive whenever they are needed. Child delivery requires only some covered space with walls on three sides. A proper room is the most suitable, but if not available, a place unfrequented by men is used. In extreme cases, babies are delivered even in fields. A secluded and covered space in the house is enough to lodge a woman for rest after child delivery.

Sometimes the cot used to deliver a child is small and worn-out. It is covered with a small bedspread called *rali* made of rags. A gunny bag may also serve the purpose. Another *rali* or blanket is used to keep the woman warm, if needed. Unlike in a modern hospital, the clothes worn during labour are not special ones. But as soon as the onset of labour is sensed, the woman changes her clothes. These are usually old and tattered ones kept specially for the purpose. As better clothes are liable to be soiled during child delivery, a woman using them is criticized for being unwise. Clothes worn during labour are called *piḍon raa gaba*, literally, clothes worn during contractions. These are later given to a *dai* or used as napkins or saintary towels.

The tools required for child delivery are usually those used commonly in every household. They do not need to be fetched from outside for the occasion. A knife or a sickle is used to cut the umbilical cord. Small folding-knives are generally available with elderly men, most of them opium addicts, who use them for cutting opium cakes. The sickle, is usually cleaned with ash or water, or may be used even without cleaning. A few people prefer shaving blades—a recent trend. A bowl of live coals is placed in the room as heat is believed to facilitate contractions. Herbs considered to be hot and heat-generating are administered, if needed. None of the above mentioned items require planned effort or time to procure. Except for medicinal herbs, which are got well in advance, everything else is already available in the house. With several people rising to the occasion, it does not take long for the items to be assembled. Thus the entire paraphernalia of child delivery involves only a few material resources.

The simple setting for childbirth and the matter-of-course attitude towards it go hand in hand. If the senior woman of the household feels less confident about handling the matter, she arranges for another experienced woman relative to stay with her overnight. Or, she is forewarned not to absent herself for long from home as she might be needed any time. Such an arrangement is usually made a few days in advance, especially if it is a woman's first child delivery. Even otherwise, the woman expert is kept regularly informed and can be called anytime as the prevailing norms do not allow her to refuse help, especially for child delivery. In fact, such an opportunity is believed to bring *punna* and is an opportunity that is foregone rarely. Refusal evokes severe criticism and disrepute. I did not come across any case of refusal during fieldwork.

A modern doctor differs from the *dai* in many respects. There are indigenous ways of keeping a *dai* informed about the pregnant woman's condition. All precarious moments are discussed intensively with the *dai*. On the other hand, the modern doctor has a fixed time when patients may come. The doctor's dealing is restricted largely to professional expertise, while the local birth expert deals in an entirely different fashion. She sees the pregnant woman as a person belonging to a particular household in the village. The *dai* also observes the patient in a total context. In order words, the pregnant woman's health is seen in the context of her household, family, caste and economic condition. Unlike medical professionals in urban areas, the local birth attendant has no fixed sehedule during which she is available for consultation. She may be approached any time during the day, and even at night, if the situation demands. As the expert attendant's or the *dai's* relationship with various households is informal, their availability for the purpose of consultancy or for attending on the patient depends primarily on personal terms. Secondly, meetings with them are not restricted only to discussions about the pregnant woman. They form only a small part of numerous matters of conversation.

The village culture ensures that the labouring woman gets expert attention when needed. The older members of the household, especially senior women, engage in resource mobilization for the event through a network of personal and informal relationships. The *dai* is paid both in cash and kind, but the payment is linked to past experiences of social relations between the two parties, sex of the baby and well-being of both child and mother. If the child is male, the *dai* is paid more. The preparations made for child delivery might appear to be casual and inadequate, but closer examination reveals that human resource mobilization is a dynamic institution assuring help when sought. Caldwell (1982: 106) rightly comments that the role of services rather than goods is rarely recognized by urban researchers.

The labouring woman assumes either the supine or the squatting position. Modesty demands that she be fully clothed except up to the knees. The *gāgro* (long skirt) is lifted up intermittently for examination of the baby's passage. Other relatives sit beside the labouring woman giving her physical and emotional care.

If a woman has an awkwardly positioned foetus she is made to stand on her head and given mild jerks to position the foetus, or a massage to guard against breach birth.[4] But she is not considered to be in any danger. She is not permitted to change sides. She remains in a supine or squatting position for hours till the baby is delivered. Efforts are made to reduce labour pain by quickening childbirth. A hot herbal soup or infusion (*ukali*) is given for fruitful contractions. Some pressure is exerted on the abdomen, but not too hard as this could damage the foetus. The umbilical cord is not cut till the placenta is out, for two reasons. First, it is believed to poison the mother, and secondly, it delays the extrusion of the placenta itself.

There is little that is unpredictable about child delivery in Mogra. Sometimes, however, there are genuine fears, especially during the first child delivery. The common expression for wishing easy delivery for a pregnant woman is both hopeful and anxious about her well-being: '*Kauḷe khēme chhūt palle vai jo*' (literally, may she happily and safely be free of the entanglement).

The matter-of-course attitude towards pregnancy and child delivery should not mean that there is no fear of maternal mortality at all in Mogra. As mentioned earlier in this chapter, seven mothers died due to complications related to childbirth; three of them in the recent past, and the remaining over a decade ago. This is much

[4] Jordan (1980) observed Yucatan midwives positioning the foetus in the uterus by massaging to avoid breach births.

lower than the 5.9 maternal deaths per thousand child deliveries in rural Alwar (a district in Rajasthan) reported by Datta *et al.* (1980). They also observed that the maternal mortality figure of three per thousand child deliveries in 1969 for all India was higher than the 0.5 for developed countries. Kohli (1977: 166), on the basis of the 14th round of NSS of rural India (1958–59), states that the female death rate in reproductive ages is 38% higher than the male death rate in the same age group.

I am unable to elaborate on maternal mortality beyond this point owing to certain limitations of my data. First, I have recorded only those cases where parent(s) were alive to report about the death of their daughters during child delivery. Six cases of maternal mortality were traced. Only in the case of Umaji's wife's death (mentioned earlier in this chapter) during her fourth childbirth, did I collect information from her mother-in-law. Her's is the seventh case. But, somehow, the fear of death during delivery rarely assumes alarming proportions. A similar attitude prevails about tetanus. (Discussed in Chapter 5.) Pregnancy and child delivery rarely call for anxiety similar to that among urban middle class couples. These are dominated by magical beliefs and cosmology. Conventional practices mobilize most of the indigenous and human resources for a smooth child delivery in Mogra.

### *Post-partum Care*

Post-partum care is well organized. Besides household members, relatives and neighbours are available for help. The special treatment given to a pregnant woman becomes more elaborate after child delivery. The rules prescribing the hours and the nature of work and rest as well as consumption of valued foods are relaxed for the *jāpāiti*. Such relaxations are considered crucial for speedy recovery. The various comforts provided to a woman are unthinkable in normal times. Their sudden availability in abundance creates a disposition which make childbirth a desirable venture for the new mother.

The *jāpāiti* avoids normal bath as her body is believed to be in a cold state. She is, therefore, given a warm sponge bath. However, the infant is bathed in warm water. The *jāpāiti* is made to sleep on a cot straight on her back with legs close to each other to heal the vaginal injury. A gauze dipped in heated sesame oil and turmeric powder is used to clean and disinfect it. The same is applied on the infant's naval, and on the cut tip of the umbilical cord. If the *jāpāiti* has abdominal or back pain, the affected area is fomented with a hot brick wrapped in a piece of cloth. A soft sash is tied around the mother's waist to regain shape.[5] She is warned not to scratch her body lest she develops striations. Women with striations are ridiculed. Younger girls hear such comments and take precautions when they are pregnant. Very few women in Mogra have the striations of pregnancy.

The effluvia is removed and the site of childbirth is cleaned. The umbilical cord is buried in a corner of the courtyard, while the remaining effluvia is buried in the household's garbage heap, usually in the cattleshed. The dung layer of the floor is peeled off and resmeared with freshly made dung and mud paste.

Though women normally do not sleep on cots during day time, the post-parturient woman always rests on a cot with the infant alongside. A small *rāli* is spread on the cot and a mini-*rāli* called *rilkiyo* on it for the baby. A gunny-bag covered with a thick layer of sand is placed under the lower part of the post-parturient woman. She lies on it with her lower body unclothed, which she covers with a bed sheet or *rāli*. She wears a *kānchḷi* (blouse) and covers her head with an *orno* (half saree), i.e. two to two-and-a-half metres of cloth used to cover the upper part of the body. The sand bed extends from the hips to the knees. This absorbs the lochia, i.e., it serves as a substitute for local variants of sanitary towels. The sand is changed daily or every alternate day depending on the need. The sand is easy to dispose of, and replace. It is available in abundance and costs nothing. In fact, it saves on rags (substitutes for sanitary towels) and water, all scarce in Mogra. Such a practice reduces material expenses, labour and other complications, thereby lightening the task for those who attend on the mother.

As mentioned earlier, a *jāpāiti* is considered ritually impure. This impurity is believed to render things in her household impure

---

[5] Both hot fomentation to relieve pain and tying of a sash on the waist are common in rural Malaysia (Laderman 1983: 158).

too. Therefore, she is secluded and not permitted to move even from her bed during the five or seven days of *hutak* upon childbirth (see Dumont 1970 on this point). The parturient woman's ritual impurity is believed to continue for at least 21 to 40 days. This belief supports the mother's bed rest while others look after her various comforts. The sand bed is used till the mother is given the first purificatory head bath, usually on the fifth day. The ritual bath can be advanced or postponed by a day or two, depending on the pressure of work on the new mother and on those attending on her. A Brahmin may also be requested to consult his almanac and declare an auspicious time for it, especially among the upper castes.

A more privileged new mother is given a massage with oil or ghee by a *dai* to relax and bring her back to the normal state. Only a few women, in Charan and Rajput castes and those of richer households in other castes, get this privilege. The majority of other women take the help of their close relatives or friends for massaging so as to avoid payment to the *dai*, while some do it themselves. The notion that body massage is desirable is gaining popularity among women of castes other than Charan and Rajput.

Many of the ailments to which the post-parturient mother is vulnerable are believed to be inflicted by evil spirits, particularly during *jāpa* (see Das 1977 for further elaboration). The community practises its own system of medicine to cure the ailment, and uses charms, libations and such other occult rituals to ward off the evil effect of spirits. A black dot on the infant's face, a black thread around the mother's as well as the infant's waist or arms, and a piece of coal on the mother's food are some of the preventive rituals practised at home.

The medication depends on the severity of the ailment. Headache, sleeplessness and restlessness are considered mild, whereas problems of lactation and hallucinations or the hearing of strange sounds are considered serious. Mothers with a history of still births, or successive infant deaths or only female issues are usually found to suffer more from such serious ailments. A body massage and an invocation to the family deity are usually considered first remedies. However, if the ailment persists, people invoke local deities or visit their common place of worship (*thān*). An oracle occasionally sits at one of the *thāns*, and is possessed by a

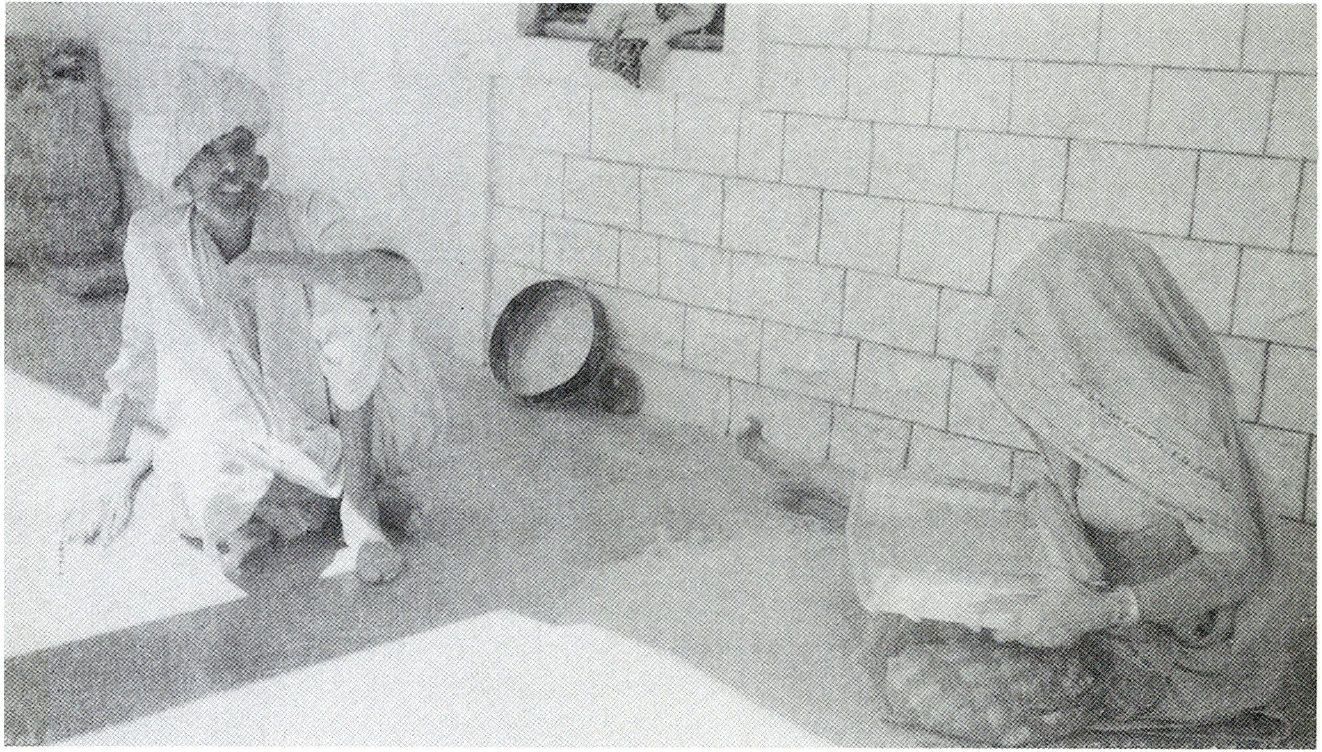

An old Patel widow, veiled and at work. Visitors rarely leave without meeting the senior-most members of a household.

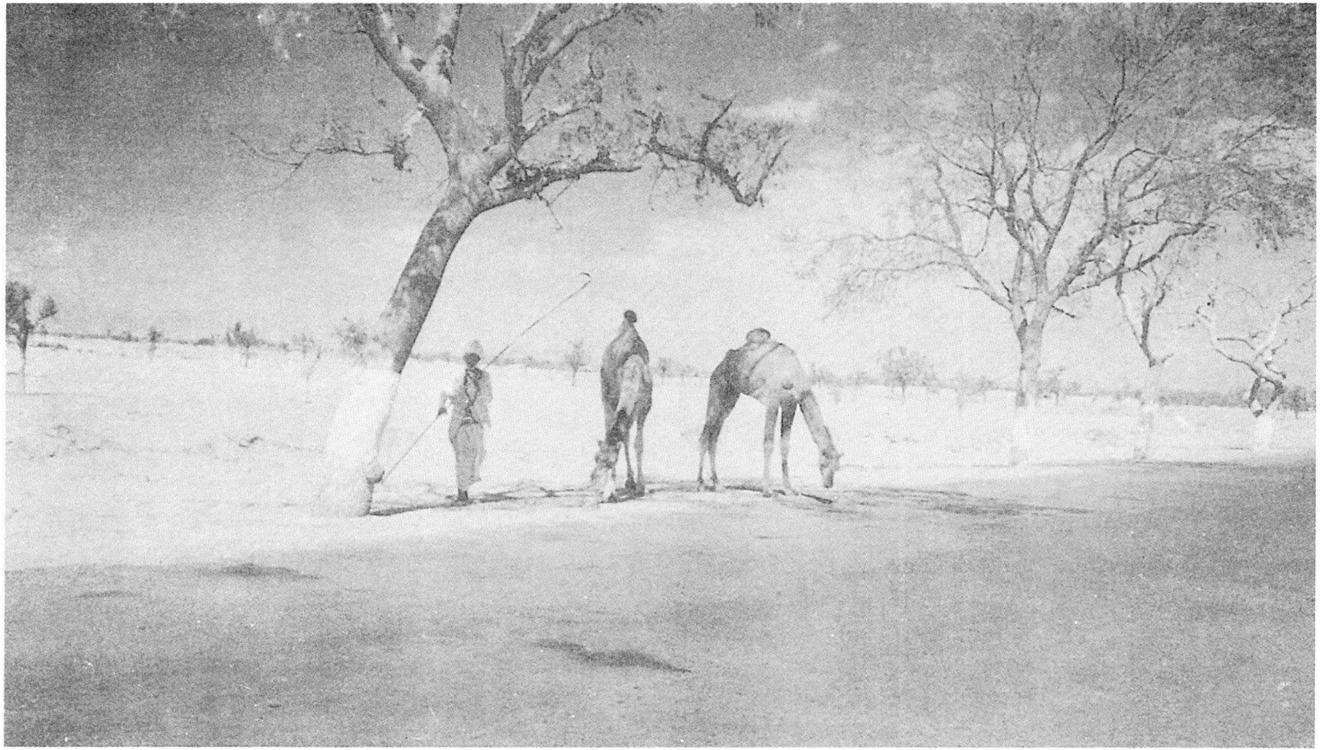

A Raika grazing his camels by the road side. Raika men have to walk long distance in search for green leaves and fodder for their cattle.

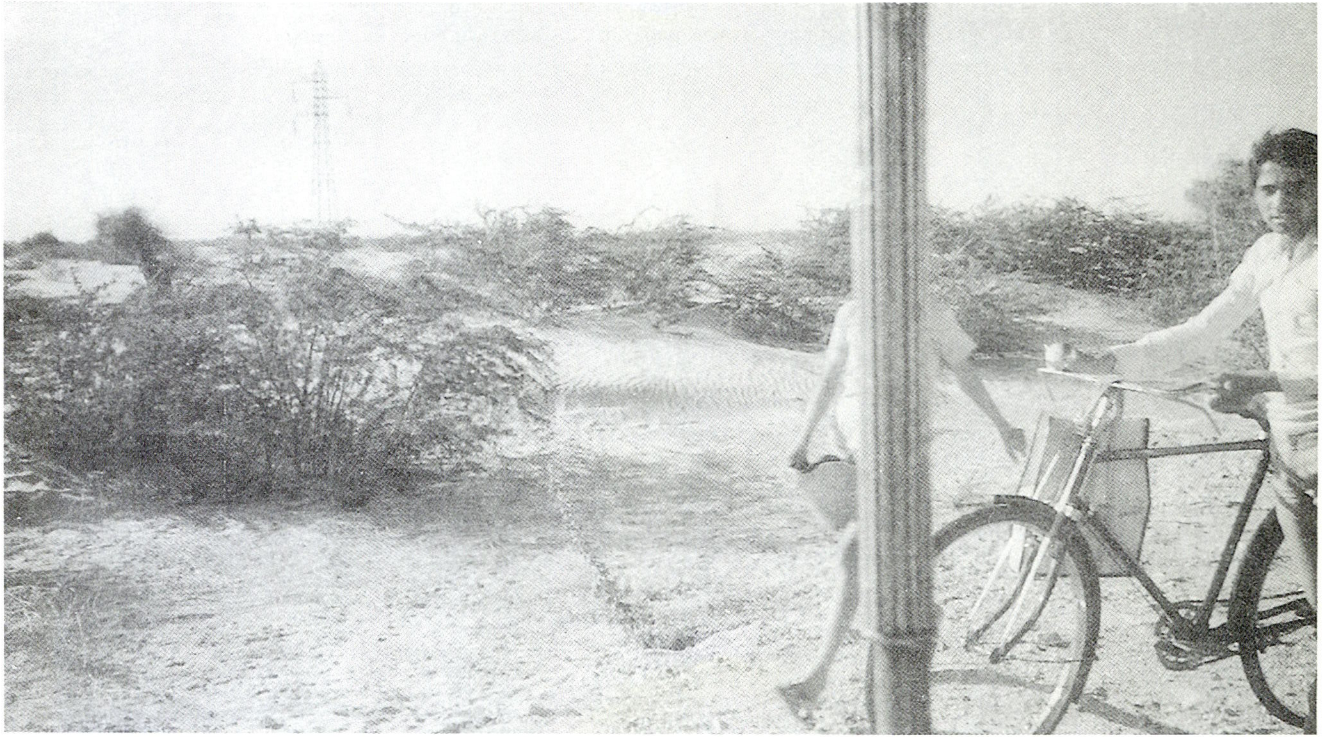

Two boys rushing home from school, get off the bicycle to get themselves into the picture.

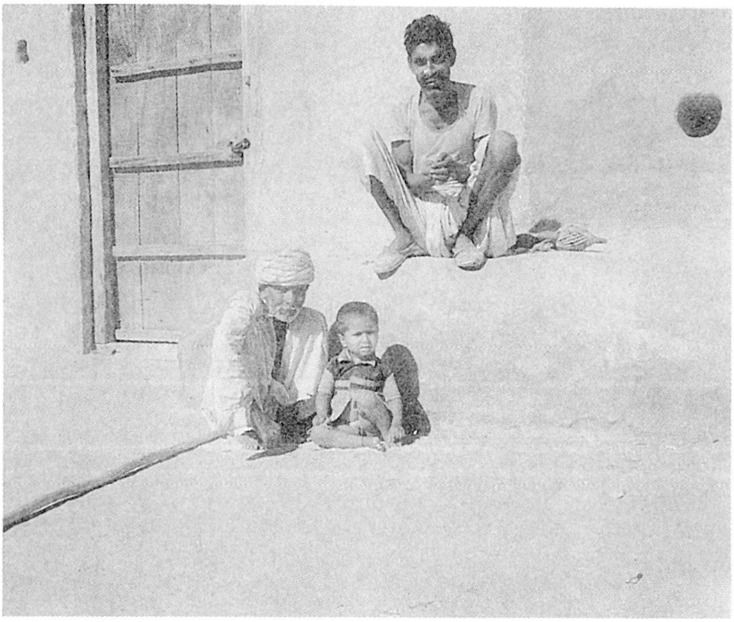

An old man with his grandson while the child's father sits at a distance. The women are away and busy with some other work.

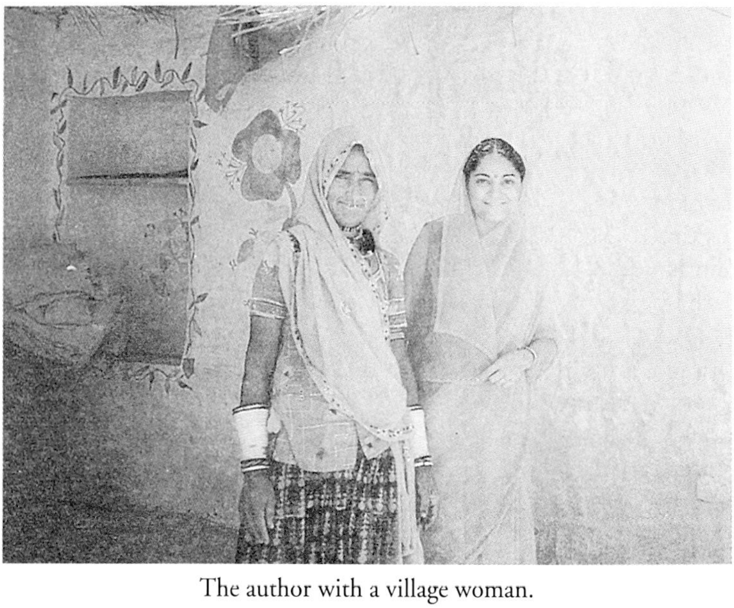

The author with a village woman.

spirit. He/she diagnoses the aliment and prescribes the remedy. If this brings no relief, then a distant *than* known for its efficacy is visited. It is believed that some of the major ailments are punishments inflicted by deities angered by an unfulfilled ritual offering or vow. Forgiveness of the deity is begged while offering libations, and promises are made to fulfil the vow soon.

One of the rituals believed to be curative is the use of amulets (*rākhḍi* and *tānti*) prepared by oracles, priests and Brahmins, and tied on wrists, arms or the neck of the ailing perosn. *Jhāḍa*, the repetitive recitation of a particular *mantra* while moving one's hand, a twig or a broom, over the ailing person to drive off evil is commonly practised. In addition, libations of sand and/or water (*dhūḍ avārṇo* and *pāṇi avārṇo*) are tried: some sand or water in a container is moved in a circular manner over the patient's body and then thrown to the left, right or both sides of the door during certain hours of the day. Besides these rituals, the elders suggest herbal treatment for curing certain ailments.

It is believed that some evil-eyed men and women in the village can harm the parturient woman and her baby in many ways. The evil eye can sometimes spoil the special eatables of the new mother, and her breast milk (the baby's only feed). Under the spell of the evil eye the food not only loses its quality but also turns harmful for the mother or the infant or both. The evil eye's attack is locally termed as *najar lāgṇo*. The ill effects of *najar* (evil eye) are neutralized by various rituals. One of them is called *lūṇ mirch karṇo*. Here, some salt and dried chillies are held in one's hand, and then circled 4–7 times over the affected mother/infant or their food. They are then thrown into fire. The pungent odour emanating from the fire confirms that the ailment is the handiwork of the evil eye. This ritual action is believed to reduce the evil eye's harmful effect on the effected person. The patient usually gets relaxed after the ritual. The *najar* is mildly feared and is generally avoided. It is warded off by secluding the parturient mother, the infant and their food from unnecessary exposure to outside people. Thus, the mother eats her *huāvaḍ* (in privacy, or only in the presence of a few trusted persons. To ward off *najar* a ritualistic gesture is made by the concerned persons. This is popularly known as *thuthko nhaukno*, mimetic spitting meant primarily to wish off evil.

All these ritual practices are organized by household members on behalf of the new mother, as her own mobility is totally restricted till the first ritual bath and usually till the *huāvaḍ* is over. Indigenous medicine is believed to take care of minor ailments of the infant and the mother. Calling a doctor is usually postponed and his help is availed of only as the last resort. Infants in Mogra are seldom taken to doctors unless they are a few months old and seriously ill.

Certain physical and dietary restrictions (*parēj*) are observed prudently. The restrictions, generally pertaining to exposure to extreme temperatures and to liquid and solid diets, rest on the common belief that the new mother is vulnerable to the severities of the winter, summer and the monsoon seasons. Even smoke is considered harmful for her eyes in the initial days, so much so that coal is brought to heat her room only after it ceases to smoke. The new mother's body is considered very tender. An excess intake of liquids is proscribed to keep her body trim and in a proper shape. The *japāiti* is given warm water only to sip and not to drink to her fill. Milk, tea, buttermilk and curd are proscribed because they are believed to be harmful when taken alongside the *huāvaḍ*. For the first few days, she abstains from routine food, green vegetables, fresh fruits (rare in any case), hot spices like chillies, etc. A *jāpāiti's* food intake remains restricted to the *huāvaḍ* only. The various precautions observed by a woman during the first *jāpa* remain the same for the subsequent ones too.

The various concessions and comforts given to the *jāpāiti* are not only an expression of society's acknowledgement of her achievement but are also meant to ensure her rejuvenation. The treatment given to the mother is independent of whether an infant is stillborn, dies soon after birth, or survives. The infant's health also receives consideration while preparing the *huāvaḍ*. For instance, some herbs are given to the mother for better lactation. Foods believed to be stale, windy, cold, spicy and sticky are avoided as they cause discomfort to the baby. In popular belief the various restrictions on the intake of liquids have no adverse effect on the mother's milk which is the baby's only feed for several months.[6]

[6] For a debate on the issue of liquid intake and its effects on lactation, see Laderman (1983: 195).

The preparation of *huāvaḍ* for younger mothers, especially during the first two or three childbirths, is a social occasion. The common practice is to invite a few women who are relatives, friends or neighbours. They along with the senior woman (in charge of provisions) of the household jointly approve the quantity of ingredients, and prepare the *huāvaḍ*. Once the work is completed, word about the amount of *huāvaḍ* prepared spreads around. If the quantity of various ingredients does not approximate to the customary norm, people disapprove of the seniormost woman of the household in gossip sessions. She is appreciated if the ingredients are in accordance with the norm. The preparation of *huāvaḍ* is organized by the mother for her daughter's first confinement and by the mother-in-law for subsequent confinements.

*Huāvaḍ* is a mother's privilege. Any arbitrary cut in quantity is actually a cut in her privilege. The quantity of *huāvaḍ* to be prepared is decided by consensus. In this manner the matter is made public. A daughter-in-law has very little ground to make allegations or accusations of being deprived of her rightful privilege. Such accusations are generally made when the demand for labour is at its peak and women do not feel strong enough to carry out the arduous tasks expected of them. Consensus regarding the quantity of *huāvaḍ* means the mother-in-law is not the sole decision-maker. Thus she manages to free herself of blame. As *huāvaḍ* is a privilege, any discrimination between daughters-in-law evokes pungent comparisons among them. A consensus saves the mother-in-law from accusations of partisanship.

## *Conclusion*

With a positive emphasis on physical work during pregnancy, the routine household activities can continue without much disruption. Nevertheless, the institutionalized practices, such as encouragement of a woman's food cravings and attempts to satisfy them, accord a special significance to pregnancy. She is considered a special person instead of being made to feel sick. The people around take care of her precarious physical condition while she performs tasks for the smooth functioning of the household and the continuity of the family line.

As an individual's identity is merged in that of the household, anything pertaining to the individual pertains to the household. The members of the household and even the larger community participate in judicious ways in the process of childbirth. The mother does not bear a child in isolation, nor does childbirth disrupt the routine chores of the household. Childbirth is an eventful occasion for the household, although it has to be physically experienced by the individual mother. Members of the kin group who eagerly await the childbirth constitute an affective human framework, which lightens the physical burden of the labouring woman.

The socialization of the girl, especially her exposure to child deliveries, prepares her to sportively endure the ineluctable labour for a desirable and obligatory childbirth that is status-enhancing. She is assured that responsible elders will take all possible care. The cultural conditioning to labour pains prevents it from being blown out of proportion. Paradoxically, the attitude of wait-and-see serves as a positive procrastination. The woman's experience of agony is partially contained through the cosmology that evaluates her character during labour pain and child delivery. Similarly, hysteria is contained by the attitude that child delivery is easier if conducted secretively from men and children.

The intimate and comprehensive involvement of birth attendants in accordance with the rhythm of the labouring woman provides an emotional cushion and an immense sense of security and care. Her being the centre of everyone's attention in an emotionally-charged atmosphere makes her participation as alive as that of others present for the eagerly-awaited tasks of child delivery. She realizes that her child's birth is as, or even more, important to others as to herself.

The participation of the household and relatives is institutionalized at the economic and symbolic levels too. The community's appreciation through rituals and gifts indicates its involvement in the woman's fertility performance. The ritual pollution is shared by the concerned households. The sharing of expenses of childbirth including *huāvaḍ* by the natal and conjugal households is an institution of intimate participation in a desirable event. Indigenous cultural practices, beliefs and restraints economize on expenditure, whether on medical expertise during and after child delivery, or hygiene, sanitation and such other comforts. The organization of childbirth through the community's informal structures hardly calls for expensive outside intervention.

*Huāvaḍ* is the best form of rewarding the mother. The social occasion institutionalized for preparing the *huāvaḍ* ensures proper care of the younger mother while she has lesser authority in the household. Every care for her recuperation substantiates the view that she has done a favour to all those concerned about the child delivery. A *jāpāiti* is recognized for her vital contribution. The rules governing labour, leisure, rest and valued food which are based on gender, seniority and kinship position are relaxed considerably for a *jāpāiti*. She gets rest, leisure and valued food, while the seniors in the household look after her comfort. These rewards are a substantial compensation for her fertility performance in a labour-intensive economy and a culture of subsistence.

CHAPTER 5

# *Child Mortality and its Bearing on Fertility*

The relationship between mortality and fertility has been demonstrated by demographers since the formulation of the theory of demographic transition. The focus here is on the infant and child mortality experiences of parents in Mogra. The main thrust is to analyse how child mortality experiences in our village impinge upon people's fertility behaviour. 'Child mortality' here includes mortality of infants (children aged less than one year) as well as of children aged one to 18 years.

Levi-Strauss (1966) states that birth and death are rich with meanings penetrating the whole of social life. Kitzinger reiterates that they are not mere physiological processes:

> To understand the meaning of birth and death, we must look for dynamic interactions between physiology, society and culture. Physiological and cultural functions are not separate, disparate entities. Eating and drinking and digestion, bowel and bladder movements, opening the body's orifices, or keeping them closed, sex and reproductive behaviour, lactation and menstruation are socially controlled physiological activities. (1982: 200).

It is in this light that the terms mortality 'incidence' and 'experience' are used here interchangeably, except that where actual mortality statistics are referred to only 'incidence' is used.

Parents' experience of child mortality is conceptualized at two levels: one, the level of actual mortality incidents as encountered by parents, and second, the perceived level, where the actual incidents are appropriated or received subjectively; in other words, at the level of meaning that the community gives to a death and of the culture-specific responses to such an event. The meaning includes people's attitudes towards death in terms of their beliefs, emotions and behaviour (for further elaboration of this point, see Durkheim 1912; Malinowski 1948; Srinivas 1952; Berger and Luckman 1967; Madan 1987). The analysis draws upon the common pool of historical memories pertaining to the experiences of birth and death of children in the village community. It focuses on the repertoire of values, attitudes and beliefs mediating between the individual and the event of mortality. The purpose of distinguishing between the two levels is to inquire as to how mortality experiences are culturally reconciled and contained. This leads us to see the bearing of the cultural repertoire related to mortality on the beliefs and practices related to fertility.

## *Child Mortality Trends*

As mentioned in Chapters 1 and 2, I have collected the reproductive histories of 713 ever married women in Mogra. Only 620 of them have attained motherhood (see Table 2.10). All those children born to these 620 mothers but dead at the time of my fieldwork are recorded as cases of child mortality. As shown in Table 2.3, the age of these women ranges between adolescence and the late eighties. The child mortality experiences of these mothers taken collectively, therefore, cover a long span of time.

I collected the information about dead children from their living mothers, fathers, or both. Except for four deaths of children aged 20 or more, all others occurred before they reached 18 years of age, i.e., before they attained legal adult status. The four cases of adult children's death are nevertheless included in our data.

Most of the cases of child death fall within the last 60 to 70 years. The earliest child death was reported by a mother aged 90 and the most recent by an adolescent mother. A limitation of such data could be that the number of deaths recorded for the past few years is high because parents tend to recall recent deaths more easily than the ones that occurred many years ago. An additional limitation is the parents' preference to avoid reporting stillbirths. Also, parents are very reluctant to recall infant deaths, especially when prodded to separate stillbirths from infant deaths that occured within a few minutes and two or three hours of birth. Despite numerous attempts, only three cases out of 111 were reported where the infant survived for an hour or two after birth. This number is too insignificant to be considered very reliable. As a result, stillbirths and infant deaths within two to three hours of birth are listed under the same category.

Child mortality was reported primarily by the mother, and if she was not alive, by the father. Other relatives and neighbours were helpful in cross-checking and giving additional information. Sex, birth order, and age of each surviving child at the time of interview were recorded, and each deceased child's age and cause at the time of death were noted. As it was not easy to get data about child deaths it had to secured through prolonged unstructured interviews. A few case studies were collected from men and women who had lost their children, siblings, and/or siblings' children, to death.

TABLE 5.1 *Distribution of mothers by number of child deaths per mother*

| *Children dead (per mother)* | *Mothers with dead children* | |
|---|---|---|
| | *Number* | *%* |
| 0 | 291 | (46.93) |
| 1 | 151 | (24.35) |
| 2 | 88 | (14.19) |
| 3 | 33 | (05.32) |
| 4 | 31 | (05.00) |
| 5 | 13 | (02.09) |
| 6 | 6 | (00.96) |
| 7 | 2 | (00.32) |
| 8 | 3 | (00.48) |
| 9 | 2 | (00.32) |
| Total | 620 | (100.00) |

Of the 620 mothers, 329 (53%) have experienced their children's death, while 291 (47%) have not. Table 5.1 shows the distribution of 620 mothers by the number of child deaths per mother. This number ranges from none to nine. Of the 620 mothers with at least one child born, 151 (24.35%) have lost that child and 178 (18.72%) with more than one child born have lost two or more of their children. As we shall see these cases are significant in the collective experience of the village regarding child mortality.

In all, 3,011 children were born to 620 mothers. Of them, 707 died (see Tables 5.1, 5.2 and 5.3). The 329 mothers who have experienced child mortality have lost an average of 2.14 children each. If the entire collectivity of 620 mothers is taken into account the average is over one child each. The death of one or two children is thus not unusual. With such a trend of mortality, parents are rarely confident about the survival of all the children born to them. In their knowledge and belief about social conditions or in their 'practical consciousness', as Giddens (1984) calls it, they are aware of the potential danger of child death.

The fear of child mortality persists in the minds of people for a fairly long period after childbirth. Deaths occur among children at varying ages. The data on child's age at death (see Table 5.2)

TABLE 5.2 *Distribution of children by age at death*

| *Age at death* | *Total children in the cohort* | *Children dead* | |
|---|---|---|---|
| | | *Number* | *(%)* |
| Stillborn or dead in 2–3 hours after birth | 3,011 | 111 | (3.68) |
| Survived for 3 hours but died within 24 hours after birth | 2,900 | 26 | (0.89) |
| Survived for 24 hours but died within a week after birth | 2,874 | 39 | (1.35) |
| Died between one to four weeks after birth | 2,835 | 51 | (1.79) |
| Died between one month and one year after birth | 2,784 | 166 | (5.96) |
| Died between one to five years after birth | 2,618 | 215 | (8.21) |
| Died between five to 10 years after birth | 2,403 | 44 | (1.83) |
| Died after the age of 10 | 2,359 | 55 | (2.33) |
| Total | 3,011 | 707 | (23.48) |

shows a high rate both in infancy and post-infancy. Of the 2,618 children who reached one year of age 215 (8.21%) died before completing five years of age. The high proportion of deaths among children up to five years of age not only reiterates the fact that a larger proportion of children die during the weaning period, it continues to remind parents that child survival is not a certainty until much after five years. Of the 3,011 children born, 707 (23.48%) have died, i.e., nearly one out of every four. This constantly reminds parents about the threat to child survival.

The survival rate of children (i.e., number of children surviving as a percentage of those born to mothers in the 45–49 age group) in Mogra is 66%. In other words, of a hundred children born to mothers with completed fertility as many as 44 did not survive. The mean child mortality is 2.60 children per mother for those who faced child death. Mothers up to 25 years of age have lost a mean number of two children each, those aged between 26 and 35 have lost 2.5 children each and those above 36 years have lost 2.8 children. Of these mothers, over 82% have lost one to three children each, nearly 16% four to six, and 2% seven to nine children (see Table 5.1). The child survival rate in Rajasthan is slightly higher than in Mogra. Srinivasan and Kanitkar (1984: 81–82) report that it was 72% in Rajasthan for the three decades up to 1981.

Infant and child deaths vary by birth order and mother's age. Demographers have generally shown U or J shaped curves in correlating age and parity with infant mortality. Jain and Visaria observe:

> . . . the infant mortality rate is found to be highest at the very young and old ages of child bearing and lower in the middle range, about 20 to 39 years. Similarly, the infant mortality rate is usually found to be high for the first order and high order births (about four and higher order parity), and low for middle range (second to fourth order birth)' (1988: 38).

Table 5.3 shows child mortality and survival incidents by birth order and sex. Of the 620 mothers, 133 (21.5%) have lost the first child. Of the 548 mothers with two children born, 139 (25.36%) have lost their second child; of the 475 mothers with at least three children born, 107 (22.52%) have lost their third child; and of the 403 mothers with at least four children born, 93 (23%)

TABLE 5.3 *Childbirth and death by birth order and sex*

| *Birth order* | *Sons* | | | *Daughters* | | | *Mothers in parity* | *children* | |
|---|---|---|---|---|---|---|---|---|---|
| | *Born* | *Dead* | *%* | *Born* | *Dead* | *%* | | *Dead* | *%* |
| 1st | 326 | 70 | 21.47 | 294 | 63 | 21.42 | 620 | 133 | 21.45 |
| 2nd | 293 | 70 | 23.89 | 255 | 69 | 27.05 | 548 | 139 | 25.36 |
| 3rd | 255 | 50 | 19.60 | 220 | 57 | 25.90 | 475 | 107 | 25.52 |
| 4th | 203 | 45 | 22.16 | 200 | 48 | 24.00 | 403 | 93 | 23.07 |
| 5th | 166 | 43 | 25.90 | 153 | 34 | 22.22 | 319 | 77 | 24.13 |
| 6th | 120 | 22 | 18.33 | 122 | 28 | 22.95 | 242 | 50 | 20.66 |
| 7th | 88 | 20 | 22.75 | 85 | 32 | 37.64 | 173 | 52 | 30.05 |
| 8th | 50 | 9 | 18.00 | 54 | 16 | 29.62 | 104 | 25 | 24.03 |
| 9th | 30 | 5 | 16.66 | 36 | 10 | 27.71 | 66 | 15 | 22.72 |
| 10th | 17 | 5 | 29.41 | 19 | 3 | 15.78 | 36 | 8 | 22.22 |
| 11th | 7 | 2 | 28.57 | 6 | 2 | 33.33 | 13 | 4 | 30.76 |
| 12th | 5 | 2 | 40.00 | — | — | — | 5 | 2 | 40.00 |
| 13th | 2 | 1 | 50.00 | 2 | — | — | 4 | 1 | 25.00 |
| 14th | 2 | 1 | 50.00 | 1 | — | — | 3 | 1 | 33.33 |
| Total | 1,564 | 345 | 22.05 | 1,447 | 362 | 25.01 | 3,011 | 707 | 23.48 |

Note: Ten cases of twins have been given the same birth order.

have lost their fourth child. The percentages of mothers with subsequent child deaths are 24.13, 20.66, 30.05, 24.03, 22.72, 22.22, and so on. The percentage of mothers who experienced child mortality ranges between 20.66% (for sixth birth order) to 40% (for 12th birth order). The data from Mogra shows relatively higher deaths from second to fifth order births. Though these figures are not large enough to make a generalization at the national level, they may be seen in the context of child bearing and rearing practices in Mogra. The practice of giving birth to the first child in the natal home and also rearing it to a certain extent there helps the mother in caring for the child. Her natal home continues to contribute intermittently towards child rearing when her second child is born. By the time she gives birth to the third child, she is considered adept at childbearing and rearing while doing other household chores. By this time her natal household provides similar support to her other siblings and she is expected to reduce her dependence on the natal home. Though she is usually helped by members of the conjugal household, the cumulative burden of rearing the increasing number of children begins to tell on her and her children's health. We have seen, for instance, that some mothers have lost more than one child at a time, as the children had a common ailment, such as smallpox, measles and diarrhoea.

Eventually, the mother gets some respite from the cumulative burden of childbearing and rearing alongside household and agricultural activities when her eldest child is old enough to look after the younger siblings. The eldest child is accorderd a special status in Mogra. The support given to parents by the first born is much appreciated. Parents look forward to such support. Hence the proverb, *mobe ghar ro thobe*, literally, the first born child is the pillar of the house. Help from the eldest child enables the mother to provide better child care to the younger ones. Thus, birth order, child mortality and mother's age should be viewed in the light of the developmental process of the household.

Child mortality is related not only to birth order but also to the sex of the child. Table 5.3 shows that though the proportion of female deaths is higher in Mogra, not every girl child is unwanted. In fact, the first girl child is rarely unwanted. Das Gupta (1987) also discusses selective discrimination against female children in rural Punjab. Our data in Table 5.3 shows that for the first birth order an equal proportion of male and female children have died, while the subsequent birth orders show proportionately more female than male child deaths.

Table 5.3 shows that of the 1,564 sons born, 345 (22.05%) have died, while of the 1,447 girls born, 362 (25.01%) have died. Visaria (1988: 91) observes that similar data at the state level shows persistent and markedly higher infant mortality rates for females than males in the northern states of India, including Rajasthan. The preferential treatment to boys, especially in feeding and medication, partly explains the lower mortality of male children. The above pattern is supported by Khan *et al.* (1983) who gathered Indian evidence indicating discrimination against daughters in the duration of breast feeding, and provision of food and medical care. Visaria sums up: '. . . the subtle discrimination against daughters by mothers, who give priority to their sons and husbands over their daughters and themselves in every respect. Such self-effacement partly contributes to the higher infant mortality of females' (1988: 92).

Of the 620 mothers, 53% have faced child death; 18% of the mothers with two children born, have lost both; over 6% of the mothers with three children born to them, have lost all three. One mother who had 14 children, had lost the first seven (to be discussed shortly). The cases where mothers have no child surviving despite a few child deliveries are sufficiently frightening for others as the fear lurks in the background. On the whole, people are more hopeful of child survival after they have had four to five children. Bulatao and Lee (1983) emphasize the need to understand the perceptions of couples regarding child survival and aptly comment that levels of child survival can be determined where sufficient demographic data is available, but couples' perceptions of these levels have generally not been investigated. We shall concentrate on such perceptions.

Of all mothers in Mogra, those 53% who witnessed their children's death are considered unfortunate by people. The mother's loss of children is referred to as *pēt balno* (literally, burning of stomach, i.e., womb). As fire burns things to ashes, the death of a child is metaphorically equated with the burning of the household to ashes. A popular remark says, *pēt ee khāli ne ghar ee khāli* and *pēt ee dhupē ne ghar ee dhuphē* (literally, both the womb and the house are empty and are squeezed to no avail). It means all labour involved in bearing and rearing of children, and the emotions and hopes invested, are wasted when a child is lost. The remaining 47% of the mothers are considered fortunate as they have escaped child mortality. They are said to have *thando pēt* (literally, cool stomach or womb). One of the several blessings senior relatives give to a daughter-in-law is *thando pēt*.

### *Social and Cultural Adjustment to Mortality*

Death is a social matter affecting the entire network of relatives. The ritual impurity affects the deceased's relatives according to the degree of affinity (see Douglas 1960 for a general discussion of this phenomenon). An adult's death is a loss to the household, the family, lineage, other relatives, neighbours and the village. People express their emotional impairment through the elaborate institution of collective mourning (*hātarvāḍo*). Relatives, friends and neighbours visit the bereaved household throughout this period. In addition, at least one member from each household in the village makes an obligatory visit (*makauṇ*) on the third day of the death to share the grief of the bereaved.

Ritual mourning (*hātarvāḍo*) is observed for a period of 11 days on the death of adult women and for 12 days for men. Besides, a longer period of *hog* or abstinence from enjoyment of good food, hobbies, bright and new clothes, ceremonial events and other pleasurable activities is observed. Members of the household and other close relatives observe *hog* at least until the passing of one of the three major festivals, Holi, Diwali and Rakhdi, in the year.

The cultural response to an adult's death is different from that to a child's. Unlike mortuary feasts held upon an old person's death, no such feast is organized nor are there any elaborate rituals performed after a child's death. An infant's death is an event in social terms but not as elaborate as that of an adult's. The duration of ritual mourning and *hog* is less for a child's death than that for an adult. Also, infants, especially girls, dying within a few days or weeks after birth rarely draw the larger community into mourning. Some of the closely related women meet the bereaved mother and other household members with a consolatory purpose. Women predominate in the customary mourning organized upon an infant's death in contrast to that for a dead adult or grown-up child. The rituals performed on the death of a child (less than 10 years of age) are much fewer and abbreviated than those following an adult's death, because a child does not acquire social personality or status like an adult.

The mourning and other rituals practised by the household and the responses of the family, relatives and the community help the members accept and adjust to the loss. The social support provides some relief to the bereaved from the deleterious effect of stress. The bereaved require sympathetic company, reassurance and care, all abundantly provided during the customary mourning period. The participation of the larger community on such an occasion provides substantial emotional support to the bereaved.

The community's participation in the process of providing relief from suffering begins immediately upon a child's death. The neighbourhood at once joins the wailing household members. It helps wash the dead body and perform other rituals for cremation or burial whichever is the case. All dead persons, adult or young, are buried among the lower castes as are dead children (aged less than 10) among other castes. While a large number, sometimes over a hundred, adult male relatives and neighbours join the procession for cremation or burial of an adult, the number attending a child's burial is usually around 20. The number may be even less in the case of a girl's death, but it is more in the case of an only son.

Soon after the cremation of a dead child, the non-lineage neighbours (believed not to be directly smitten by grief) bring simple food for the bereaved household. It is upon their consolation and insistence that the bereaved accept food. No food is cooked in the bereaved household on the day of death. A similar practice is reported by Srinivas (1952) among the Coorgs and by Dube (1955) in Shamirpet in south India. The bereaved household is helped to gradually resume its routine life through institutionalized participation of the community in numerous ways in the mourning process.

When the mourners visit the bereaved house, they sit next to of the grieving family and relatives. All of them then weep together. Subsequently, the visiting mourners shift a few feet away from the bereaved and talk to them consolingly. They mostly recall other unfortunate, untimely and unnatural deaths in the community, primarily with the intention of showing that the bereaved are not the only ones to have suffered, and to enable them to be strong enough to take death as an irreversible fact. The religious ideas of fatalism and karma are frequently invoked.

Members of the wider community express their proximity to the bereaved household just when they have suffered. The group expresses its bond by weeping. Mourning is the impression of loss felt by the group and brings individuals together into closer relations. Durkheim (1912) showed how through piacular rituals mourning provides a sensation of comfort which compensates for the original loss, and how celebrations have the object either of meeting a calamity or else merely of commemorating and deploring it. Malinowski (1948) similarly emphasized how the function of funeral ceremonialism is to reaffirm the fundamental meanings of society and solidarity in the face of the ultimate threat. Berger (1969) elaborates that death not only poses an obvious threat to the continuity of human relationships but it also threatens the basic assumption of order on which human society rests.

In Mogra a continuous dawn-to-dusk wailing for at least the first four days goes on, in which one's fellow villagers as well as friends and relatives from the neighbouring villages participate. During the 12 days of mourning, except on Tuesdays and Sundays, believed to be hard days (*ākro vār*), the bereaved weep, wail and remember the deceased. Mourners keep coming throughout the day. Women visitors wail loudly, in a standardized manner, upon entering the street. In response, the mourners in the house raise their wailing pitch. The weeping, wailing, lamenting, holding each other, etc. continue. These sessions are renewed intermittently.[1] The wailing is heard in the neighbouring streets. The overall atmosphere is dismal. The neighbourhood suffers the loss indirectly during the period of ritual mourning. The bereaved are constantly surrounded by mourners lest grief overtake them in loneliness. Stroebe and Stroebe (1987) suggest that grief is resolved more rapidly in those societies where there is family and community support—it promotes quicker recovery after a loss by death. These are social resources for problem-solving.

Living and dying are thought to be interrelated experiences in society. In addition to one's hope in the ability to replenish, there are several other aspects of cosmology that are invoked to enable the grieving to adjust to the loss of their near and dear ones. Fatalism and the theory of karma constitute two strong pillars of

---

[1] All the visiting mourners (wailing in a standardized manner) appear to be almost equally affected by a death, but actually many of them rarely feel the chagrin expressed. As a member of the moral community, one is constrained to weep. It is a ritual attitude and respect for custom. Srinivas (1952: 110) aptly distinguishes ritual mourning from grief at the death of a person. Even though the parents of a deceased infant may actually be steeped in deep sorrow, the period of ritual mourning is rarely prolonged, especially if the infant is only a few months old.

people's cosmology to adjust to several life experiences, death being one of them. They commonly invoke terms like *lek, kismat, jog, bhāg*, etc. (literally, what is written on the forehead, destiny, chance, luck). It is believed that one's *lēk* is inscribed by God even before one is born. One is destined to realize and enact the divine inscriptions. It is common for all people to refer to one's *kismat* or *bhāg* in the event of both joy and sorrow. This belief should not, however, imply that people do not work hard to achieve socially-cherished goals in life. They do work hard in most spheres of life. Fatalism simply comes to their rescue when the goals are not met or when something unexpected throttles their efforts. It is one's moral duty to take death as given, or, as villagers say, to accept it as fore-stamped on the parents' *bhāg* (fate), and to attribute its cause to a supernatural power whose command has to be obeyed.

A similar passivity is found in peoples belief in the theory of karma and rebirth. It is an active part of their common consciousness that one's ascriptive status and life-achievements depend on one's performance in the previous incarnation. The same logic is extended to the relationship between parents and children. The children are in this respect seen as having been related to the parents in some form in their previous incarnation. A child is said to be born to its parents in this incarnation either to pay off debts it owed them in some past incarnation or to recover its dues.

Certain practices symbolically help contain the infant and child mortality tribulations of parents and close kin. We have analysed in Chapter 3 the aspect of social onomastics pertaining to the birth order of children. Another aspect deals with child death. A set of names are given to children whose parents have experienced high child mortality in their reproductive career. The commonly assigned names are Ladhu or Labu (found), Bheeka, Manga (begged/borrowed), Natha (anchored), Dhaḷa, Dhagḷa, Uka, Dhuḍa, Reta or Phoosa (sand/dust/garbage), and Koja or Bhoonda (ugly). These names express three different forms of parental anxiety for child survival: (1) the found or borrowed, (2) the anchored and (3) the worthless. Children with such names reflect the unfortunate initial fertility experiences of their parents. The names meaning 'found', 'borrowed' or 'begged' indicate that the parents' status is that of mere custodians. By implication they are not supposed to be the owner-parents of the child. The child is considered to be owned by someone else, usually God. The names meaning 'anchored' indicate the plight of unfortunate parents who have tethered the child to prevent its escape from this custody. Names meaning 'sand', 'dust', 'garbage', etc. connote worthlessness of the child so that it is not subjected to the evil eye either by ordinary human beings or by evil spirits. Garbage, sand, etc. have few claimants. These names convey a symbolic message that they are worthless and should remain abandoned to their parents.

People perform some death-averting rituals also. Often a child is weighed with grain which are then given away as alms. Very often parents or other household elders vow to give alms to Brahmins, Saads, and Saamis, and to feed cows, birds, etc. for a child's survival. They also vow to offer deities sweets, grain, etc. if a child's death is averted. These vows are akin to those made during labour for successful child delivery, as mentioned in Chapter 4.[2] Parents are also known to carry the dying child to a temple and leave it there so that it can survive under God's benevolent care. If it happens to survive, it is rarely taken back. The child then becomes a part of the temple community. The parents feel happy that their child is alive even though it is not growing up with them. I found two such cases in a temple in a neighbouring village (cf. Madan for similar practices among Hindus in Kashmir).

### *The Dead and the Living*

Frequently a child's death is negated symbolically. This is done by giving a new infant the name of the child that has died. The parents then consider themselves fortunate, and say, 'It has come back to us,' or 'It had been taken away by mistake and has been returned, we are destined to be its parents.' They feel that one child's death has been evened out by the birth of the other. Malinowski put it crisply, 'He who is faced by deaths turns to the promise of life' (1948: 47).

[2] Vows to offer sweets, money, etc. to deities, to give alms, and to feed cows and birds are believed to be efficacious acts of religiosity. Such vows are made for averting deaths, including those of cattle. For instance, a sick cow or calf is left at certain temples to survive under God's care.

People believe in the existence of a deceased's *jīv* (spirit/soul, not necessarily ghost) in the atmosphere around. The spirit, once it leaves the body, is called *jīv*, and dying is referred respectfully as the giving up of *jīv* (*jīv diyo* or *jīv dei diyo*). It is further believed that for 11 days (before the final death ritual is performed) the *jīv* hovers around, and is usually considered to have an influence, neutral or benign, but rarely evil. Although the *jīv* is neutral, it has to be kept at bay. The *jīv* is not considered to be a ghost (*bhoot/prēt*).

It is believed that the *jīv* of a person dying anytime between early teens and middle age (during which several desires may be unfulfilled) may turn into a ghost. In other words, untimely or unnatural deaths, called *kāchi maut* (literally, unripe deaths), are thought to retain in the world of the living, the desires of the deceased's *jīv* which could return as a ghost or a malefic spirit capable of harming the living. The dangerous and evil ghosts are believed to reside near crematoria or on certain trees, which are to be avoided during certain hours of the day, and at night. A ghost tends to possess and trouble people. It is to be overpowered and controlled through occult rituals. It is a *jīv* that has not attained *gati*. Attainment of *gati* transforms the *jīv* into a *pitri* (ancestor) or a benign spirit. The numerous rituals performed till the twelfth day of death are meant to turn a *jīv* into a benign spirit. For assured *gati*, the ashes and a few bones of the deceased are immersed in the holy Ganga, called *Gangāji mein ghālna* (to immerse in the Ganga), and a mortuary feast is organized upon return from the Ganga (cf. Atal 1968 for a similar practice in a south Rajasthan village). Upon attainment of *gati*, a *jīv* severs all its worldly ties and ceases to be harmful to the living. It is then revered and occasionally offered food and prayers.

Apart from being a ghost or *pitri* (ancestor), a *jīv* can exist in another form. In some cases a *jīv* refuses to attain *gati* and yet does not turn into a *bhoot* (ghost). Instead, it becomes a *pittar* (manes). Such a *jīv* insists on space in its erstwhile house. This is revealed through a *thān*. Arrangements are made to ritually bring in the *jīv* and assign it a place of worship akin to that of a household or local deity. The *jīv* is often referred to by the name of the deceased. A *jīv* placed back in the house for worship is called *pittar*. Its presence is usually considered benign for the household and, in some cases, for the larger community as well, unlike a harmful ghost.

> One of Dharamji's sons, Sona, in his late teens, died in a road accident. He was made a *pittar* on his (Sona's) insistence. Now his benign spirit possesses Dharmaji's second son once a month. The house becomes a *thān*. A large number of believers gather around the *thān* on that day every month.

In other words, a *pittar* continues to be alive in people's mind. It is some consolation to parents that they can make supernatural contacts with a deceased child who is spiritually alive.

The refusal to recognize a child's death is accompained by the equally emphatic unwillingness to recall such deaths. Most of the parents refuse to recall their dead children. They are often touchy about the issue, particularly when directly questioned. When I asked mothers about their child mortality experiences, some of them suggested modestly and evasively that the dead need not be recalled, and others lost their temper and were outraged. Those who had assembled around the respondents expressed their dislike for such recall. They usually commented: 'Those who have gone are gone. Don't mention about them. What can we do about them now? We don't remember such matters. Of what avail is their memory?' It was a trying time to collect data on this issue (see Appendix 1).

### *Causes of Child Mortality*

As already mentioned, information on causes of child mortality was collected along with that of birth order and sex of the deceased children. For a precise study of the causes of death, biomedical professionals would be required. Since I do not possess the expertise I have depended only on the diagnoses, imaginary or real, as perceived and reported by the respondents. The primary purpose here is to understand people's perceptions of child mortality. The socially-defined concepts of illness and disease suffice largely for the present purpose (see Djurfeldt and Lindberg 1976: 20–26 for a review of the strengths and weaknesses of the approaches of 'biomedicine' and 'ethnomedicine'). Disease is not only suffered, endured and treated but also explained and talked about. Disease concepts are verbally labelled and readily communicable (cf. Frake

1973 for elaboration of this issue among the people of Mindanao). A person fairly conversant with a culture understands the name and the etiology of disease rather easily. People's reporting of the causes of death included allopathic, ayurvedic as well as folk theories.

When people assign causes to their children's death, some of them are clearly natural causes or body ailments, while others are believed to have been inflicted by malefic spirits, witches, ghosts and demons. People strongly believe in the efficacy of witchcraft and sorcery. Most of the evil spirits, devils, demons, etc. are considerd harmful, especially for children's life and health.

The causes of death of 707 children are classified into five categories in Table 5.4. Since the causes are derived primarily from reasons provided by people, the categories lack a uniform biomedical criterion. Different kinds of ailments are reported as causes of death. For instance, a very common ailment, fever (*tāv*, i.e., pyrexia of unknown origin) is a major killer. Ninety five deaths were reported as caused by it. It assumes dangerous connotations and is considered a major illness when it prolongs for a few months, as death results. Therefore, fever is categorized as a major physical ailment causing death. On the other hand, boils and pain in the finger (caused by an infection) are considered minor ailments. Deaths from such ailments are fewer than from prolonged fever. Thus, between two ailments causing child deaths, one is considered a more potent cause than the other.

Of the five categories into which the concepts of disease are classified here, the first category constitutes what people consider to be major physical illnesses, i.e., serious disorders of the body. These include protracted fever (*tāv* or *bukhar*), tetanus (*tauṇaun*), typhoid (*nikāḷo*), diarrhoea (*dustaun*), tuberculosis (*tibee, T. B.*).

No reason was assigned to 123 deaths. In most of these cases, the child had died even before the parents were able to figure out the illness. Also, some of the parents did not wish to discuss the illness as it was agonizing for them. They preferred to feign ignorance of the cause to ward off the tragic memory. The parents reported either evasively or ignorantly the causes as 'don't know', 'sudden death', or 'some illness', and could not recall even the symptoms. Similarly parents and other senior household members

TABLE 5.4 *Distribution of dead children by cause of death*

| *Cause of death* | *Children dead* | |
|---|---|---|
| | *Number* | *(%)* |
| I. Major physical ailments: | | |
| Prolonged fever (*tāv*) | 95 | (13.4) |
| Typhoid (*nēkāḷo*) | 28 | (5.7) |
| Growth failure (*hūkṇo*) | 26 | (3.9) |
| Diarrhoea and/or vomiting (*dastaun/ultiyoṛ*) | 26 | (3.9) |
| Heat-stroke (*loo*) | 24 | (3.3) |
| Tetanus (*tauṇaun*) | 20 | (2.8) |
| Polio and paralysis (*lakwo*) | 7 | (0.9) |
| Maternal mortality (*tābar avṇūn hō*) | 6 | (0.8) |
| Jaundice (*piḷiyo*) and pneumonia | 6 | (0.8) |
| Tuberculosis (*tibee*) | 5 | (0.7) |
| Tumour and blood vomiting (*gaunth* and *cancer, khūn ro*) | 3 | (0.4) |
| Accidents: on road, burning, drowning, snake bite (*aeru*) | 7 | (0.9) |
| Sub total | 268 | (38.0) |
| II. Supernatural inflictions: | | |
| Smallpox (*mata*) | 42 | (5.9) |
| Measles (*ori*) | 41 | (5.8) |
| Eaten by a witch (*dākaṇ*) | 26 | (3.6) |
| *Ratva* (Affected by menstrual blood) | 13 | (1.8) |
| *Uparlo* and *lila piḷa* (some curse) | 8 | (1.1) |
| Chickenpox (*achhabaḍa*) | 6 | (0.8) |
| Sub total | 136 | (19.2) |
| III. Minor physical ailments: Headache, pain in finger, boils, escabies, giddiness, backache, etc. | 69 | (9.7) |
| IV. No reason assigned | 123 | (17.3) |
| V. Birth-related accidents | 111 | (15.7) |
| Total | 707 | (100.0) |

were unable to mention the specific causes of death of 111 infants. In these cases, the infants were either stillborn or had died within a few hours of birth. Very minor ailments were the cause of

9.7 per cent of deaths. Although supernatural afflictions are common explanations, only 136 (19.2%) deaths were believed to have occurred from them. The largest number of deaths, 268 (38%), were caused by what were believed to be major physiological diseases (reported in biomedical terms).

Of the 473 deaths for which causes were reported, the major ones were: prolonged fever—95 (20%); measles and chicken-pox—47 (10%); smallpox—42 (9%); typhoid—41 (9%); growth failure—28 (6%); diarrhoca—26 (5.4%); attack by witches—26 (5.4%), explained locally as 'the child was eaten by *dākaṇiyon*'; heat-stroke—24 (5%); and tetanus—20 (4.2%).

As regards deaths 'due to attack by *dākaṇ* (witch)'—certain elder women living in the village are perceived commonly as 'eating' away infants and children. The *dākaṇ* symbolically eats away the child's liver or sucks its life from the body. People fear and avoid meeting such women. The existence of witches is common in rural Rajasthan. They are supposed to operate upon the viscera of their victims through looks or incantations and make them succumb (cf. Tod 1920: 88, 1051, 1113 for this belief in Rajasthan during the 19th century). Chuni, an old woman, recalled how particular her mother-in-law was to prevent her children being seen by a *dākaṇ* who lived in the back street. Such women are believed to have a secret knowledge of turning into cats at night to eat away infant livers.

There are, in fact, a large number of cats in the village. Eatables and newborn infants have to be specially guarded against stray cats. The ill effect of cats is reflected in the light-hearted comment addressed to naughty and foolish children by elders: 'Where had the cats gone (when you were born)?' The implication is 'Did they not take you away, you the worthless?' The child is reminded that he/she is so undutiful that cats should have taken it away after birth. In other words, the elders' constant watch of the child during its neo-natal stage has been a waste, because the child is good for nothing.

Rajasthan in general has a high infant mortality rate. But, both in Mogra and in Rajasthan, unlike most other states in India, tetanus is not the cause of the maximum number of child deaths. It ranks as one of the 20 top killer diseases in India as a whole and in most other states, but not in Rajasthan. Instead, pneumonia, prematurity, typhoid, diarrhoea and others in descending order are major killer diseases (see Registrar-General, India 1983: 28, 33). I have not explored this intriguing fact further.

Certain illnesses are believed to be inflicted by supernatural forces, such as a curse by a deity, the onslaught of a demon, a devil, or a witch hovering around at certain odd hours, and the pollution of a new born infant by a menstruating woman (*ratva*). In addition, the death of infants because of premature birth, low birth weight, anomalous birth, or the death of two or more children one after another within a few months after birth etc., are not assigned any medical reasons. They are perceived as effects of some curse inflicted on parents and/or the child. Measles (*orī*), smallpox (*māta*) and chickenpox (*achhabaḍa*) are believed to result from the wrath of the angered female deity, Mataji (literally, mother). For the latter three inflictions propitiation of the deity is regarded as the only remedy, and no medicine is administered to patients, except abstinence from certain foods. However, for all other 'supernatural' afflictions some 'medicine' is usually administered along with propitiation of deities or the ritual warding off of malevolent spirits.

For some other deaths parents and other elders are unable to give any specific reason either in terms of a serious physical illness or a supernatural affliction. Instead they describe some of the symptoms of the child's ailment (in biomedical terms) prior to its death as a cause. In other words, they provide a localized, symptomatic diagnosis as the cause of death. These include minor ailments such as pain in finger, giddiness, backache, boils, swelling, stomach-ache, refusal to have milk or food, and suspension of weeping. These are categorized as minor ailments in Table 5.4. People believe that all supernatural inflictions are caused by unfavourable stars, or by poor karma. People try to cure an illness and avert death in numerous ways. But when their attempts fail they blame their fate and karma and try to reconcile themselves to the unfavourable attitude of deities.

Although people offer causes and explanations of deaths, they believe that ultimately death follows God's will. In other words, a person dies only when God wishes. They explain that disease, illness, or accident is only a pretext and not the real cause of death, because God does not take upon Himself the responsibility for it (*Ram matē nee lea*). People support their belief by asking: 'Why, can the doctors not avert death?' They answer by saying: 'God is the supreme commander of life and death. Death comes if it is destined to come, irrespective of whether a person is attended or unattended by medical experts. There is no escape from death if that is God's dictate. Uncertainty of life and death is the other side of the certainty of God's will.'

If a mother loses two or three babies successively in a few months of birth, the death is associated with the deleterious properties of mother's milk. Such mothers are admonished by household and other elders to discontinue breast-feeding. This in turn makes the infant more vulnerable to death. The infant's death and the consequent suspension of breast-feeding reduce the spacing between births. New born infants in such cases are weaker. The mother also becomes debilitated, thereby reducing the infant's survival chances. Births and deaths at quick intervals form a vicious circle in which such a mother is trapped. Not only the mother but her entire household is seen as suffering from a 'supernatural curse', or the influence of a malefic spirit.

### *Cases of Excessive Child Mortality*

As noted in Chapter 3, children bring honour and prosperity to parents. Accordingly, their death amounts to loss of honour and prosperity to parents. The feeling of being unfortunate and economically disadvantaged due to high child mortality is also reported for Kashmir by Madan (1987) and for Africa by Caldwell (1982). Untimely deaths (*kāchi maut*) of young persons and children are particularly shocking.

Three women in Mogra have lost 4–9 infants each within a few days to a few months after birth. The birth intervals ranged from 11 to 18 months. Most of them were exceptionally feeble. Two of the three mothers have each only one child surviving after several pregnancies and childbirths. The third mother has lost all six children born to her but cherishes a faint hope that at least one child would survive in the near future. All the three women are pitied by their relatives and neighbours. The women themselves feel helpless and cursed. They blame their poor fate (*phaura lēk*) and poor karma (*phaura karam*). The socio-economic status of all the households is below average. Their husbands are the lone earners for the household. For most part of the year, these women are occupied with child bearing; they are physically indisposed and too feeble to work during pregnancy and post-parturition. Child survival would have changed the picture of their households.

Child mortality experiences are not restricted to the death of one's own children but also include those of others in the community. Those who participate in sharing the grief of the affected ones are equally aware of the potential danger of child mortality. The collective fear is experienced both on the event of death and on other occasions, when the dead are recalled not only by those parents who have experienced a high incidence of infant and child mortality but also by those who have had no first hand experience of it. Thus, the anxiety and uncertainty of children's survival besets parents uniformly, irrespective of their individual experience of child mortality.

Fear of child death lurks not only in the minds of parents who have experienced it first hand but also in those who have not. Not having experienced the death of one's own child does not erase completely the fear of child mortality from a person's mind. Cases of parents who have lost grown up children, particularly all the sons, are concrete proof (for others in the village) of the constant threat of child mortality and its consequences.

> Jamni, a Patel widow in her seventies, has reverted to Mogra from her conjugal home in another village. She has been living in Mogra for the past two decades. She lost her only son when he was in his early thirties. Jamni's widowed daugher-in-law resorted to *nāta*. She remarried elsewhere within a year of widowhood, leaving behind a two-year-old daughter. Jamni had only one married daughter to call her own. For more than a decade now, Jamni is pitied by all people. She has to perform all tasks herself, whether they are the ones performed usually by children, adults, men, women and old persons. Jamni's case is frequently recalled to pacify bereaved parents. People say, 'She is just killing the miserable time for which she is destined to live. Such a life is not worth living, but God does not give death to her. She is a born sufferer (*Jalam ree dukhiyaraṇ hae*).' People frequently wish that she had more sons. Her relatives and neighbours are eyeing her fields and property. They very often put pressure on her to part

with some of it, saying, 'For whom do you need land? You have no one to pass it on to.' The worst time is when she falls sick. Despite being self-sufficient and not dependent on others for any economic or physical requirements, Jamni somehow carries on. She is very strong. There are very few people in the village as old and who work as hard.

But being active in old age is a secondary virtue. Of paramount value for the aged in the village is having a large family with several adults and children in the household to ensure sufficient leisure coupled with social life and opportunities for pontification. In the absence of adult children and grandchildren, an aged person, however active, is only pitied.

Bhanwari, a Jat widow in her fifties, popularly known as Gangu's mother, appeared to have aged rapidly within a few months of her 22-year-old son Gangu's death by typhoid. On seeing me enter her house, she stopped milking the cow half-way and burst out emotionally: 'Why can't God give me death? He is cruel. He has taken away my son when it was actually my turn to leave the world,' she cried.

She could not explain why she was destined to be so unfortunate, 'I had borne five sons and two daughters. But only one boy and one girl grew up to be adults. All others passed away in childhood. The daughter is married. The widowed daughter-in-law has gone away after Gangu's death, leaving me all alone in this world. Look at these pots and pans. I had acquired them over all these years for Gangu and his family. Each of them gives me a sting as I see them. There is no one to live in these rooms. Everything is gone with Gangu. What have I achieved in this life?'

Gangu's mother's tale is that of an unfortunate, sonless widow. The proverb symbolically conveying the emptiness of a house and womb is truly applicable to her. Such tragic cases of the death of a grown up son only reinforce the traditional logic of having several sons.

Amiya, a Charan widow in her fifties, has faced a similar crumbling of the household and herself. After the marriage of all her three daughters, her 15-year-old son died. Two years later, her husband also passed away. Later, her husband's brothers had their eyes on her large property. They did not even allow her daughters to reside with her on a regular basis. Adopting a daughter's son was not an easy task. Her husband's brother—customarily the most rightful claimant—would not let this happen. Amiya

> turned hysterical at times. She has become more suspicious of people and more quarrelsome, her neighbours observe. Her major fear is, 'Who will look after me if my property is snatched away?'

Having land and other property for a comfortable livelihood are not at all enough for a sonless widow. Her deceased husband's agnates keep a constant vigil on her property and wait for her death to grab it. The absence of a son makes it difficult for married daughters to stay with their aged parents.

> Kacku, a Patel widow, is the lone survivor of a family that consisted of two households and 20 members. Death was at its worst in her case and she has felt it all the time. She is haunted by memories of the five rooms in her large house that were once crowded with people. Memories are galore though each room is a vacant structure of bricks, walls and roof with no men, women or children. Two years back, even her *kāki-haoo*, classificatory mother-in-law (husband's father's brother's wife) died. Till then the two widows had lived together for several years, as both had lost almost all their household members. Five years ago her only surviving son who had been affected by polio died. She had two sons and three daughters. Both the sons' speech and legs were impaired when they reached around nine years of age. Each suffered for a few years and died. Kacku had to make arrangements to send the dead bodies of her sons to the crematorium. She lamented that if the misfortune had not struck her, the sons would have carried her dead body to the crematorium. Later she wanted one of her married daughters to come and join her. But the lineage members protested and did not let her fulfill her wish.'

Kacku's case is more horrifying than that of Gangu's mother, Jamni and Amiya. She has seen the deaths of 20 members of the household since she joined it upon marraige in her teens. The worst aspect of her hair-raising case is the opposition of her lineage members to her bringing in a *ghar jamāi* (permitted, among Patels, customarily). She could then live with one of her daughters, her son-in-law and their children. Not every parent suffers from the deaths of so many children, however.

### *Parent's Response to Child Mortality*

A mother's experience of several childbirths and child deaths has been interpreted in varous ways. Bhatia (1963) argues that early fertility, and malnutrition increase the possibility of infant deaths, which in turn leads to increased pregnancies at smaller intervals, weaker mothers and more infant deaths. Agarwala (1970) gives a typical demographer's explanation without going into any of the conditions that may be responsible for numerous births and deaths. He looks at it from a side opposite to that of Bhatia's, and states that mothers who give birth to a large number of children not only lose a large number of them but the proportional rate of child mortality is also high. It appears from Agarwala's comment that if women produce more children, they lose more too. But this is so only on the face of it. A deeper look at fertility experience in Mogra shows that mothers have more children when they lose more. Wyon and Gordon (1971) also observe that women who lost only one child or none from the first three to six children born alive did have fewer subsequent children than corresponding women who lost two or more children.

The fear of child mortality lingers on in parents' minds not only during their offsprings' childhood but even later. As we have seen, over 50 of the 707 children died after crossing the age of 10. People usually feel the need to provide for unfortunate child mortality incidents and for the resulting insecurities. Tilly (1978), and Cain (1981) have also shown a close relationship between high infant mortality and high fertility in some Asian and African communities. Caldwell and Caldwell (1981) summarized how both individuals and societies attempt to enhance chances of child survival in tropical Africa. In Mogra too people provide a margin for child mortality. It has terrified some of the couples so much that they have returned to normalcy only by making up for their loss by producing several children. This gives them the hope that some of them would survive.

> Mangli, a 50-year-old potter woman, gave birth to 14 children in all, one of whom was stillborn. She had to work more than other women of her age. Despite being senior in age, she has not been able to attain the status of a mother-in-law. Of her 14 children, the first seven died. Her eighth was then the only surviving child. She then had seven more children, and considered herself fortunate enough to see them all surviving. Mangli fails to understand why people put a stop to fertility. Her own experience of losing one child after another has shattered her so much that she sees meaning only in a continuous bearing of children. Besides,

> her own name (Mangli, i.e., begged) suggests that she was a much-desired child of her parents. Her parents' and her own grim fertility experiences have contributed to her indomitable conviction in high fertility.
> Gomti, a 35-year-old Saad woman, gave birth to 10 children, four of whom died. The deaths made her very insecure till she had six surviving children. The extent of her insecurity was so much that she did not wish to stop bearing children. She said, 'Having had 10 children by now, I'll have only two or three more. And who knows how many of them will remain before my eyes (surviving).' The same fear haunts Gopi, an old Harijan woman who lost five of her 11 children.

It is clear from the above cases and from Table 5.1 that people resort to high fertility when child mortality evens out their earlier fertility achievements. It is wise to have more children when their survival is not assured (cf. Djurfeldt and Lindberg 1976: 196 for an account of the risk of child death). People prefer to have many children so that a few may survive. Srinivasan makes the same point: 'Many studies carried out in recent years in India and other countries both at the macro- and the micro-levels reveal that period and cohort fertility measures are strongly and consistently associated with mortality levels.... The linkage of fertility to previous experience of infant and child mortality is one of the established facts of demography' (1986: 173–74).

Couples not only experience the mortality of their own children but also observe and recall the loss of their siblings' children, and those of other relatives. This has been found in other parts of India as well. Mahadevan *et al.* (1981) report the same for all groups—Muslims, Harijans, and upper castes in Andhra Pradesh. Namboodiri (1986) argues that sequential fertility since couples decide about it in accordance with their experience over time. There need not, of course, be a one-to-one correspondence between mortality and fertility. The hiatus between child mortality and parents' fertility is bound to surface when life chances are not always assured. Such a hiatus is also reported by Kunstadter (1984) for Thailand. Heer (1972) in his Taiwan study reports that women who perceive the chances of survival of children up to the age of 15 years as 95% and above , have fewer births after the birth of the second child than those who perceive their survival as 85% or less. Pebley *et al.* (1979) in a study of Guatemalan women found that the experience of child mortality, and the death of one's own children and that of siblings are strongly and positively related to the desire for additional children at parity three and above.

In Mogra, the unfortunate cases of untimely deaths are recalled from time to time. Even cases from neighbouring villages are discussed. All such experiences form a part of collective memory. They are cited as the worst examples of parental misfortune. An occasional wish is expressed: 'Even enemies should not face such a misfortune.' The threat of child death in Mogra is so contagious that even those couples who have not lost any children are aware of the threat.

The fear of mortality in general increases particularly during the outbreak of disease and drought. Certain forebodings of disaster (symbolic indicators) are believed to bring misfortune, especially death. For instance, deaths on certain days of the week, the whining of dogs and the roar of the wind are sensed as signals of death. Tuesday and Sunday are believed to be hard days (*ākro vār*). A death on a hard day is believed to be a premonition of another within a week. Such instances are recalled by elder men and women in the village. I saw five deaths (of two children, two old men, and one woman in her early twenties) occurring within a period of 10 days in Mogra during the fourth successive year of drought in 1987. The warning bells are symbols of danger perceived collectively, and the belief is strengthened intermittently as happened during the 1987 drought.

### *Fertility Response to Fall in Mortality*

The persistence of high fertility remains a demographic puzzle despite the fall in mortality in most developing societies. Mogra is no exception. General mortality and child mortality have decreased in India as a whole including the state of Rajasthan (Jain and Visaria 1988: 28–29). Srinivasan and Kanitkar (1984: 81–85) observe that Rajasthan once experienced very high mortality rates but they have declined dramatically during the past 10–15 years. Visaria (1988: 96) points out that infant mortality rates in rural Rajasthan declined from 152 in 1973–5 to 118 in 1982–4.

In Mogra, the older mothers (above 35 years of age) have lost more children than their younger counterparts. On the other hand, with the fall in mortality rates over the past few decades, the younger mothers' experience of child survival has increased. But fertility in Mogra continues to be high. It has not declined proportionately with decreased mortality. There is no mechanical link between mortality and fertility. The discrepancy between fertility and mortality trends may be understood better if people's perceptions are taken into consideration.

The social norms of fertility and the repository of experiences of past and present fertility and mortality continue to influence people's behaviour in favour of high fertility. Although younger parents have, on an average, experienced lower child mortality, they were occasionally reminded of high child mortality till the recent past. Senior members in the household and the neighbourhood, and other relatives recall their own and others' child mortality experiences. We have already discussed the numerous occasions when people's child mortality experiences are recalled vividly. The fear of child mortality continues to persist in the minds of the younger parents too.

The decline in mortality from a very high to a relatively low rate is not sufficient to neutralize the fear of mortality. Parents are seldom assured fully of their child's survival. The persistence of high fertility can partially be explained by the lingering fear that not all children born to younger couples are sure to survive. The infant mortality figure of 118 per thousand live births in 1982–4 for rural Rajasthan is too large to be ignored. The mean child mortality per young mother (up to 25 years of age) is two children, and three for mothers above 35. The cultural values, norms, symbols and rituals mediating fertility continue to persist in society. The cultural values and norms are deeply internalized and are not amenable to change in a mechanical fashion and immediately in accordance with any fall in infant and child mortality incidence.

Nevertheless, a few couples have attempted to curtail their fertility at an early age. They have done so, however, only after achieving the prescribed minimum fertility, namely, two sons and a daughter. The trend towards accepting modern fertility control methods is emerging albeit not at a pace equal to that of the decline in mortality, as we shall discuss in detail in Chapter 7.

### *Conclusion*

The analysis of infant and child mortality experiences both at the factual and the perceptual levels highlights the social and cultural mediations through which infant and child mortality is contained and overcome. The reduced mortality, however, has hardly attenuated the veracity of rituals and cosmology that enables people to accept and explain mortality. The common pool of historical experiences and folk wisdom expressed in the associated values, beliefs and norms has a bearing on people's adjustment with and response to infant and child mortality.

CHAPTER 6

# *Indigenous Modes of Fertility Control*

Demographic literature is replete with observations of an inverse relation between certain attributes of modernity and family size (Thompson 1929; Notestein 1945; Coale and Hoover 1958; Leiberman 1980, Srinivasan 1986). These attributes are industrial economy, higher female literacy and gainful employment of women outside the household. They form a framework wherein couples are expected to acquire attitudes favouring fertility reduction. These attitudes are supposed to be rooted in the couple's ability to make decisions and exercise control. The image of a modern couple derived from this construct is one of rational beings who actively confront the conditions of life. They do not passively accept the dictates of the conditions of life and regulate their fertility with a view to organizing life in a way as to control it better. Thus the modern couple consciously curtail their fertility rather than leave it to the natural course.

The above argument is also used in demographic studies pertaining to traditional social settings, typically underdeveloped and rural societies with high fertility. The rural couple is portrayed in this literature as having little control over the conditions of their lives and as governed in matters of fertility more by impulses than by rationality. Their fertility follows an unhindered course, without any conscious intervention on their part (Lorimer 1954; Howell 1979; Wilson 1984). Many studies explain the high fertility of traditional societies in terms of certain values and attitudes towards women, their low status, rural economy and a veritable lack of individualism.

Demographic studies focusing on cost-benefit calculus of fertility behaviour also corroborate the same argument (Thompson 1929; Becker 1960; Mueller 1972; Leibenstein 1981). They try to show that couples in modern, urban, industrial societies rationally calculate the costs and benefits of having children and deliberately curtail their fertility, while couples in traditional societies tend to have more children. The modern couple is contrasted with the traditional, such that the former subscribe to a rationality controlling fertility, while the latter reproduce as long as their fecundity permits.

There is no society in which people reproduce to their bio-logical capacity, notwithstanding the very high fertility of the Hutterites (Caldwell *et al.* 1987). Handwerker (1986) highlights the futility of the thesis of 'natural' fertility. On the other hand, some demographic studies (Enke 1966; U.N. 1974; Endres 1975) go to the extent of saying that in India high fertility is a reflection of copulation being the only means of recreation among rural people. There is nothing to do except go to bed after dark (see George's 1976 discussion on this issue).

That these studies betrary a skin-deep understanding of the reality of fertility behaviour becomes clear as soon as an attempt is made to take into account the sleeping patterns (discussed latter in this chapter) and leisure activities in traditional societies. These studies ignore the immense richness of local institutions of entertainment, recreation, relaxation, fun, merry-making and gossiping, not to mention well-developed folk arts, music and songs. These aspects of rural life can be known only through an in-depth knowledge of people's lifestyles and world view. Unlike modern, industrial societies, the insulation of 'labour' from 'leisure' has not yet come about in rural societies like Mogra. Labour and leisure overlap here. Recreation, fun and frolic are knit into the working of society. In addition, there are several festive occasions when leisure predominates labour.

I hope to show in the present chapter that the image of rural people's fertility behaviour is erroneously formulated and empirically unwarranted. Much of demographic literature is scantily informed of social norms and structural conditions that enforce lowering of fertility in traditional societies. Nevertheless, a few demographic studies have recognized the prevalence of controls in primitive/traditional societies. Carr-Saunders (1922) observes that pre-modern societies control their own fertility. Heer (1964) reports that Indian-speaking communities in parts of Andean countries practise voluntary control of fertility. Douglas (1966) describes how various primitive communities maintain their population by controlling it with the help of their customary beliefs and practices. Smith (1977: 142–3) has discussed traditional mechanisms of fertility control in Japan. Bloch (1908: 696), Firth (1963), Benedict (1970: 165–180), and Polgar (1971) describe population regulation in primitive societies. Freebeme (1964) mentions the practice of fertility control in traditional China.

Some references of traditional mechanisms of fertility control in India have also been reported. Mandelbaum, while handling the material on human fertility in India, is struck by the realization that, 'There are also certain forces favourable to birth limitation, although information about them has not been abundantly available or systematically presented and has been overshadowed by a good deal of misinformation' (1974: 13). Similarly, Wyon and Gordon (1971: 236, 311) conclude that the Khanna villagers, in their traditional ways, practised appreciably more birth control than originally supposed. Djurfeldt and Lindberg (1976: 194), Unni (1979: 67) and Caldwell *et al.* (1984: 190–193) refer to the practice of traditional fertility control in south India. I shall also document how people in Mogra are governed by definite indigenous modes of fertility control and not guided merely by an unrestrained biological instinct.

The focus here is on the norms of fertility trajectory and how it is regulated during a couple's reproductive career. What are the beliefs and practices behind the organization of nuptial space, family size, birth intervals, and indigenous techniques adopted for fertility control in Mogra? How do social norms regulate and control fertility, both in terms of a person's stage in the life cycle and the number of children born? How do norms proscribe procreation after the socially optimum number of children have been born and are surviving, and what are the related beliefs and practices?

How do customary practices of fertility control support fertility regulation and control mechanisms?

### *Pregnant Grandmother Complex*

We have just noted a few studies that report on the social disapproval of the grandmother continuing to bear children in India. Chandrasekaran (1986) goes to the extent of stating that in contrast to several other cultures, including the west, it is only in India that both men and women believe that procreation should cease after a person advances in age, especially when one's children are old enough for procreation. But such disapproval is found in other societies as well. Caldwell and Caldwell (1977) and Caldwell (1982: 141) elucidate the proscriptive pregnant grandmother syndrome prevalent strongly among the Yoruba in Nigeria.

In Mogra, a grandmother ceases to bear children. Attaining an advanced stage in one's fertility career makes a couple eligible for suspending procreation. The norms proscribe the time when a couple should opt out of having a baby of their own and have babies from their children instead. Ideally parents are expected to abstain from or to give up sexual life once their children are married. By the time a woman achieves the status of a successful mother, i.e., has a few grown up children, especially sons, she is aged around 35 years. This is when her sons and daughters are to be married, i.e., their *muklāwo* is due. As age at marriage is low, the *muklāwo* of a girl usually takes place by the time her mother is around 35. This is the time she is likely to become a mother-in-law, a high position for a woman in the status hierarchy of her household and the family. At this stage she acquires the prerogative to put an end to her fertility. Thus, giving up procreation usually results from a combination of three factors: (1) achieving the socially optimum number and sex proportion of children, (2) advancing in age, and (3) attaining the status of a mother-in-law as a consequence of her son's or daughter's marriage.

Women rarely procreate after crossing the age of 40. The few mothers who have had children after this age had either lost many of their earlier children, or were without a son, or had not attained mother-in-law status. Those parents who pay little heed to the sexual norm after the age of 40 are ridiculed as well as frowned upon. The pregnancy of old women or mothers-in-law is subject of fun and humour. They are criticized for being over-indulgent in their sexual relations at an age when most older couples relinquish it. A few of the commonly made comments are: '*Budāpa mein ee jak nee paḍē* (there is no sense of satisfaction even in old age);' and '*tābar ne maiet hātē kāna jaṇe bakariyon, larḍiyon jyoon* (how unbecoming of parents to procreate alongside their children like goats and sheep).' If an old couple continues to engage in sex even without any bearing on conception, it provokes a lot of gossip and latent derision. Comparable observations have been reported from other social settings in India (U. N. 1961: 137, 143–56; Mathen 1962: 44; Opler 1964: 218; Gould 1969; Caldwell *et al.* 1984).

It is worth recalling here the discussion on the norm of patrivirilocality in Mogra. While in a small proportion of cases all or most of the married sons continue to reside with parents, in a majority of cases they secede from the joint household. In which case, at least one son continues to live with the parents. In other words, old parents are never left all alone in the house. The household composition and sleeping arrangements are also such that it is difficult for an old couple to have sex unobtrusively. The elderly members and grown up children sleep in common places like the courtyard. In summer, older men generally sleep on cots spread on the street or in an open space in the house like the courtyard, where other boys also join them. Senior women sleep in a space adjoining the courtyard, at a little distance from their husbands. If old men sleep on the street, women place their cots in the courtyard amidst other members of the household. Young daughters-in-law usually sleep each in a separate room, a shed, or a corner not directly visible from the courtyard occupied by others. The young husband joins his wife at night when others fall asleep. In this sleeping arrangement it is not difficult for adult members to sense the absence of the elderly. Their absence seldom remains undetected. If the usual sleeping spaces of senior spouses are found vacant for some time during the night, it becomes a subject for gossip. In no way do sex relations of the elderly remain a secret for long.

The socially expected family size and the normative fertility trajectory are so deeply internalized by parents that it is reflected even in their symbols and language. This is particularly so in the pattern of nomenclature. (This is one more aspect of social onomastics discussed in Chapters 3 and 5.) The elderly parents' unwillingness to have children is revealed in the names assigned to those born after the parents have had the socially optimum number of children of both sexes. Names meaning 'undesirable' are given to such children. They are indicative of the parents' acknowledgement that they have tampered with social norms and did not really want the child. The names indicating the parents' unwelcome attitude to their later children are Madi (one who has barged in), Aaichuki (enough of coming), Santi (peace/quiet), Santos (satisfaction/complacency) and Dhapuri (satisfied/full/complete). These names are not assigned to the first few children. They imply that although parents have accepted the infant they were keen not to have it in the first place.

It is also worthwhile to mention the sex bias in names. If a son is born after it is unbecoming of parents to continue procreation, he is rarely given such a name. In other words, a son is not named as unwelcome even after the couple has achieved the socially optimum number of children. Nevertheless, once a woman becomes a mother-in-law, any child is unwanted, irrespective of the child's sex.

### *Fertility and the Developmental Process of the Household*

The set of norms crucial to ending further procreation are observed not simply because they are internalized by the members themselves. Certain conditions circumscribing women's life also instil in them a desire to stop bearing further children. These conditions converge in a married couple's life usually when their children are married, i.e., in the culmination phase of their fertility career.

A newly-married adolescent bride's interest in the conjugal household increases gradualy with the passage of time. Whether she establishes her nuclear household or continues to live in the joint one, she gets enmeshed into numerous and overlapping role sets in the household as well as in the network of relatives. The household and neighbourhood support decreases gradually with additional childbirths, i.e., the post-parturient mother is thought to be adept at taking care of herself and the infant. Even the care, concern, and comfort provided by the household to the parturient mother ceases to be the same as that provided during the first few childbirths. The celebrations and applause wane in their intensity. Gifts from relatives and neighbours decline. Additional children do not enhance the older couple's status or authority substantially. A couple with two grown-up sons and a daughter gets only a marginal increase, if any, in their status with the birth of additional children. At this stage the woman has a strong desire to put a stop to her fertility.

With the progression of the household, the status and responsibilities of the mother also get transformed. Many women secede from complex households to set up nuclear family households usually after they have had two to three children. These women then have the major responsibility of running their own households. The pressure of work is greater on them. In such a situation they themselves prefer to reduce the duration of post-partum rest. Usually, childbirths cease to be an attraction as the period of post-partum rest is curtailed by the mother herself, and status enhancement is only marginal, unless child mortality has taken the toll of the children born earlier and evened out previous achievements. By this time, the woman's interest in the household becomes more entrenched. She feels that the expenses of *huāvaḍ* as well as the loss of work days during post-partum rest cut into household resources. Earlier, as a young daughter-in-law, she stole brief intervals during routine arduous tasks under the pretext of baby care and baby feeding, but now her interests lie more in hard work. With such a change in household interests and consequent enhanced status, frequent pregnancies and child deliveries hamper the woman's interests as well as routine activities.

Similar conditions are also encountered by those women who do not secede from the complex household and continue to stay with the parents-in-law. These women have the advantage of being helped by parents-in-law in matters pertaining to neighbourhood and community obligations. At the same time they have to frequently receive and entertain many more guests than in simple households. Invariably parents-in-law represent the household in such matters, while the younger couples make the requisite arrangements.

> Kacku, the youngest of three daughters-in-law, and the only one living with her parents-in-law, rarely has to suspend her household work for the sake of several social and community obligations, such as gossiping with guests, visiting another household in the village to mourn a death, or visiting a relative in a neighbouring village under a kinship obligation. Her mother-in-law does all this. She representes the household to mourn a death in and outside the village, pays 'get well' visits to ailing neighbours and relatives, attends ceremonies of childbirth and other obligatory social meetings. She sits and gossips with guests, while Kacku engages in routine household work and cooks for the guests. But both her elder sisters-in-law who live in separate households, have to make the obligatory visits by suspending their household work. Similarly, in extending hospitality to guests, her sisters-in-law have to combine household work with attendance on guests, while Kacku shares with her parents-in-law the responsibility of hosting them.
>
> Kacku's husband rarely has to suspend his work because his father graces most of the obligatory social occasions. Doongarji, Kacku's father-in-law, receives most male guests and gossips with them. He represents the household when an obligatory mourning visit is to be made. He does the same on several other social visits. Of course, Kacku and her husband Kera are not detained in the house. They attend several ritual and festive events. As in all joint huseholds, there exists a division of labour in Doongarji's household. But Kacku's husband's brothers living in nuclear households have to suspend their household work whenever social obligations demand. The latter will get some respite when their children reach adolescence and share many tasks.

Around this stage in life, i.e., the culmination phase of the fertility career, a woman foresees the need to accumulate resources for her growing children's marriages and for the mortuary feasts of her old parents-in-law (all sons share mortuary feast expenses irrespective of their separate or joint residence).

Despite the presence of traditional support institutions, senior women feel crushed under the weight of repeat pregnancies and child deliveries. It is not uncommon to hear their experiences of pain and anguish. In most of these cases, they desire earnestly to seek respite from continuous reproduction.

> Thirty two-year-old Vaski, a Patel woman, entered her conjugal home at the age of 16 upon *muklāwo*. Four years later she had her first child, a daughter, who is now 12 years old. Vaski moved out of the conjugal household with her husband and four children to live in a separate house 12 years after *muklāwo*. After seceding, she had two more children. That is, three sons and three daughters in all. After seceding, she had two more children with a gap of about two years between each of them without using any contraceptive. Despite following the same sexual behaviour as in the past, she was surprised that the gap between her last two children was only a year. Four of her six children are very young, and looking after them takes a lot of her time and effort. It is quite a bother, although her eldest daughter helps her in various ways. Yet, Vaski's strength is giving way. She confided that she wanted to avoid childbirth since the past one year. 'Three daughters and two sons were enough, I thought. But another came recently. I tried to find out about contraceptives but could not get exact information on any. Someone suggested a herbal remedy, but the associated taboos to be carefully observed put me off. I have not tried any contraceptive yet. I dread another conception.'

Women's unwillingness to have more children finds expression in their constant crabbing and irritable behaviour. They often prefer to stop procreation even before attaining the status of mother-in-law, especially after they have had the socially optimum number of children surviving.

> Sugan, a Charan woman aged 27 and mother of three sons, said, 'I am tired of reproducing. Even after the second son was born I did not want any more. Going on reproducing every alternate year is being like goats. Goats don't have to nurture and discipline their young ones. But humans have the bother of looking after their children. None of my three sons wants to stay at home even for a minute. They frequently pick up quarrels with children when they go out and also get hurt. I am really fed up with them. I can't even go out everytime to check or monitor them.' (Being a Charan woman, she observes *purdo* and does not move out of the house unless she is assured that no men are around). 'But my husband and mother-in-law have no sympathy for me. My incessant requests for sterilization have fallen on deaf ears.'

The interest a young mother has in controlling fertility is not always shared by others, especially by the mother-in-law and the husband. Consequently, her crabbing is rarely heeded.

> Maggi, a 30-year-old Patel woman and mother of three daughters and a son, narrated her predicament: 'All through the nine months of pregnancy I lie down like half dead. I have no energy to work. I dislike eating, and feel nauseated all the time. But some household work has to be done. I have to cook for the children and their father. Fourtunately, the eldest girl can fetch water in a small pot that takes care of the thirst. The entire household faces numerous inconveniences while I carry the baby (foetus). My sickness ends only with child delivery. Only after taking some *huāvaḍ* am I able to regain strength and revive the household. But the work of an infant's mother is always done in bits and pieces. I have to attend to the infant. I am convinced that an end to my regular pregnancies can save me from looming death. But my husband wants one more son. He says, "what is the assurance that our only son will survive? Try to be wise and wait till we get the second son. You may sterilize after that". He does not understand my misery and fear.'

Although the mother may feel exhausted with recurrent childbearing and prefer to put an end to child deliveries, she has to contain her impatience for a few more years in the hope of another son (furthering the progression of the household) before she is considered too senior to reproduce. The above cases show how mothers with a few surviving children, including sons, genuinely prefer to put an end to procreation, although their desire may not be fulfilled immediately. The predicament of these mothers shows the interplay between societal norms and individual desires. Her ability to control fertility arises out of her position in the social situation in the household and outside (cf. Lealock 1986). By the time she attains the ability to control her fertility, she already achieves the socially optimum number of children, particularly sons. It is the interplay of factors such as motherhood and assertiveness accruing from a substantial period of stay in the conjugal household that makes a woman bold enough to put a stop to her fertility.

### *Social Management of Birth Intervals*

In Chapter 3, we have seen how a new couple follows social norms regarding the onset of fertility, i.e., maintaining the socially prescribed minimum duration between marriage and first childbirth. There also prevails what may be called a socially prescribed fertility career which regulates the couple's initiation into the reproductive career, the long drawn process of bearing the socially optimum number of children, and putting an end to procreation. An important mode of indigenous fertility regulation is the prevalence of social practices that favour a certain interval between births. It is possible to identify a few such practices which may be distinguished from each other in terms of the manner in which they affect couples. First, there is a norm that parenthood should not result before at least two years of marriage. Secondly, the institution of breast-feeding, including prolonged lactation increases the duration of amenorrhea. Thirdly, according to a widely prevalent attitude, the lactating mother is seldom extended a nutritively rich diet during the entire course of lactation. Such nutritive deficiency also accounts for prolonged amenorrhea. Fourthly, sexual abstinence is prescribed during certain periods.

In Mogra, the average birth interval (locally called *hoe*) for mothers who have given birth to more than one child is 27 months. Mothers with only one child are excluded from the calculation of birth intervals. Stillbirths as well as live births are taken into consideration for the present purpose. However foetal wastage is not included. Of the total of 3,011 live births, only 27 cases of foetal wastage were reported. This, however, is different from that reported in the west (Potter 1963: 158) where a hundred pregnancies usually produce about 88 live births, 10 miscarriages and two still births. The low figure in Mogra may be explained partly by people's sense of modesty in recalling and reporting miscarriages and abortions. Only 7% of mothers had a short birth interval of less than 22 months, while a tiny fraction (3%) of mothers had a long gap of over 52 months. For about 90% of the mothers the *hoe* ranged from 23 to 52 months, and of them, for a large majority the *hoe* was 23 to 32 months. A gap of about two years between two childbirths is considered the minimum in Mogra. Those having children within one year of their *muklāwo* are ridiculed. Wyon and Gordon (1971: 158, 168–9) report similarly for Khanna villages in Punjab where two years of breast-feeding prevents early birth of the next child.

In the absence of these and other customary practices, the birth intervals may not have been what they are. They would have been reduced. This was predicted by Potter and Parker (1964) about American women. The women who had regular intercourse without contraceptives had the probability of conceiving within three months of the last childbirth. Birth intervals in Mogra show that despite rare use of contraceptives, most mothers' *hoe* is about two years.

One of the institutions that spaces births is abstinence from sexual intercourse during certain periods. Post-partum abstience is one such, the period ranging from two to four months. It is believed that if a couple violates the norm, it would adversly affect their ritual purity and health. A woman is believed to be continuously impure (especially for sex) for a period of 41 days after childbirth, although the extent of impurity sub-sides after the ritual head-bath on the fifth day. Sexual abstinence is strictly practised during this period. However, the socially expected period is two months after childbirth. Non-observance is reprimanded by household elders and other close relatives.

All women deliver the first child at their natal home. The confinement lasts for two to four months, separating the spouses till the new mother returns to her conjugal home. Even after the proscribed duration of two months, the frequency of intercourse remains minimal for some time. The manner in which the sleeping space is organized diminishes the privacy of couples. The newborn and the young mother are usually under the constant care and protection of elderly women in the house. Constant protection is crucial because the infant is vulnerable to the bites of cats and rats infesting many a house. In such a situation even verbal communication between the spouses is reduced considerably. The employment of post-partum sexual abstinence in many societies, especially in sub-Saharan Africa, as a deliberate attempt at family limitation is reported by Caldwell and Caldwell (1977) and Page and Lesthaeghe (1981).

Other occasions for short-term abstinences for couples include menstruation, sickness, mourning and religious ceremonies. Separation of spouses for a few months at a stretch in the initial years of marital life is also institutionalized. This is done through the custom of a married girl living in her natal home for longer durations and making fewer intermittent visits to her conjugal house, more so among castes other than the upper ones. Similarly, as mentioned earlier, the first childbirth is postponed by norms maintaining a time gap between *muklāwo* and childbirth. Usually the prescribed duration of such an interval is at least two years. But in certain cases it stretches even up to 5–6 years. The mean interval is three and half years (see Table 2.10 for women's age at first childbirth.) If a couple happens to violate the norm and has a child in less than two years after *muklāwo*, people consider it indecent and an affront to their sense of modesty. The cultural values proscribe women from showing any initiative in sexual matters. Such a restraint is also reported from other parts of India (see Gould 1969, Poffenberger 1969, Rao and Mathen 1970; and Nag 1972).

Another important practice accounting for regulation of birth intervals is the mode of breast-feeing. In Mogra, mothers breast-feed their infants on demand. People consider mother's milk as the only vital nutrient for the infant. This belief is so strongly ingrained that infants are not even given water for a considereable duration, i.e., for two or three months, if the child is born in summer, and for four to five months, if in winter. It is believed that giving water to an infant can cause it a throat infection, called *gaḷo paḍno* (literally, falling of the throat). Mother's milk is considered so crucial that even if she has no milk due to some ailment or post-partum exhaustion, the infant is nursed by a wet relative. If a mother has less milk, some herbs are prescribed for her to facilitate proper lactation. When the infant is around eight months old, milk, other than the mother's, is gradually introduced. For about seven to eight months the infant survives solely on mother's milk.

Supplementary feed such as milk and cereals is administered around the age of eight months. Semi-solid and other foods are not specially cooked for the infant, except that it is given *chūrmo* (mashed *roti* with ghee) or *dūd roti* (mashed *roti* with milk). A piece of *roti* may also be given to the infant to nibble at, and keep it occupied, leaving others to do their routine chores. Cereals are not fed as long as mother's milk can sustain it. This is primarily for two reasons. First, it is believed that cereals cause diarrhoea in the initial stage. This causes discomfort to the infant and inconvenience to the mother and other household members, because it involves constant changing and washing of nappies. This task becomes more tedious in a situation of water scarcity. Secondly, there prevails a strong belief that if an infant is fed cereals its stools stink badly. It is also believed that mother's milk is the only feed that leads neither to diarrhoea nor to malodorous stools. Thus elders find it convenient to delay introduction of cereals and prolong the infant's dependence on mother's milk. As the infant grows, its demand for breast-feed increases, and as a result the frequency of feeding goes up. It is not uncommon to feed such an infant at an hourly interval. This practice of breast-feeding on demand has an important bearing on prolonging the anovulatory period considerably. Reduction in breast-feeding increases fertility by reducing the period of sterility among women. This is reported by Mosley (1977) and Alexander (1984) for Java, Wolf (1969) for late 19th and early 20th century Mexico, China, Algeria, Vietnam and Cuba, and by Laderman (1983) for Malaysia.

The weaning of an infant from breast milk and supplementation with cereals generally leads to the onset of the mother's menstrual cycle. But breast-feeding is not discontinued till the next conception is discovered. And if there happens to be no further conception, breast-feeding continues for five to six years for the last child. The significance associated with breast'feeding can be understood from the fact that if an infant dies very early, the previous child is again put to suckle in a conscious attempt at avoiding quicker conception. Senior women of the household and the neighbourhood usually encourage this practice while the mother is in grief. They justify their attempts at putting the elder child to suckle by saying that without doing so the grieving mother would conceive too early.

Another important factor accounting for the prevailing pattern of birth intervals is under-nourishment of the lactating mother. The much coveted *huāvaḍ* lasts only for a few weeks after child delivery. Beyond this period a new mother is considered healthy enough to continue to lactate without any extra nutrition. Nevertheless, whatever the mother eats is believed to have a direct influence on the infant's health. For a few months, the post-parturient mother observes certain restraints in food intake. She avoids food items believed to have strong hot, cold or sticky properties such as milk, rice, bananas and leftovers from earlier meals as they are believed to adversely affect the infant's digestion.

Overall the lower nutritional intake by women coupled with continued breast-feeding leads to the physical weakening of most mothers. This state is described as *chūngaḍ nee hadē*, literally, 'suckling does not suit.' Thus, because of continued under-nourishment most mothers have long anovulatory periods. There is hardly a case where a mother's menstrual cycle resumes before 10 months of childbirth, save in those cases where the infant dies within a few days of birth.

Why was fertility high despite longer birth intervals in the past? Firstly, as we have seen in Chapter 3, high fertility is advantageous to couples in numerous ways. Secondly, a high rate of child mortality, as discussed in the previous chapter, rarely, gave older couples the confidence to stop procreation as soon as they achieved the socially minimum number of children. But in recent times, as noted in the latter part of chapter 5, an incipient trend is emerging in favour of fertility control soon after couples have the socially optimum number of children. The three cases of young mothers, viz., Vaski, Maggi and Sugan, described in this chapter highlight their confidence about child survival and consequently their desire to stop procreation. In their fertility behaviour the older husbands and wives provided for child mortality.

### *Emergent Changes in Practices Regulating Birth Intervals*

Having examined the social practices influencing birth intervals, let us turn to recent variations occurring in them. Differential birth intervals are found among mothers belonging to different age cohorts. In other words, the average spacing between children is not the same for the older and younger mothers in Mogra. The older mothers (aged 35 and above) have longer average spacing between children than the younger mothers (aged less than 35).

The shortest average gap between births observed in Mogra is 12 months. Four young mothers are represented in this category. There is no older mother with such a short birth interval. Similarly, a larger number of younger mothers are found in the next spacing interval of 13 to 22 months.

Changes are emerging in the social values and institutions influencing birth intervals among younger couples. Education and urban exposure have some influence, rather incipient now, on traditional institutions. First of all, a major change can be seen in the value of modesty. The younger spouses now dare to identify themselves with one another openly rather than show mutual indifference before senior household members and other relatives in the initial years of marriage. Younger couples occasionally express an overt interest in each other's affairs. Older people express their concern about the younger couples' lack of modesty (*hanko*, hesitation) in recent years. Most of the elderly contrast their own behaviour with that of the younger ones. For instance, in the past, the newly married man visited his wife's natal home usually five or six months after *muklāwo*. This period coincided with some festival, usually Diwali. But of late, many younger sons-in-law visit their wives even before the completion of the prescribed period, and they often do this secretly, though it rarely remains so for long. Early first visits are becoming a part of the changing ethos of marriage. Many older persons openly express their disapproval of it.

> Shivji, an old man, commented annoyingly about his son's visit to his in-laws' within three months of *muklāwo*. 'These boys have no shame (*lāj*) at all. They lack even basic common sense to feel how their parents will react to it.' Shivji's friend Chimji, who was sitting beside him, also endorsend the comment and said: 'Even the air seems to have changed. The younger generation behaves without heed to the sentiments of their elders. They are always restless to meet their wives.' Vijaji had a point to make. He stated in a reflective moment: 'When we were young, we never had the moral courage to take the initiative to visit our wives' parental homes on our own. In fact, our parents used to pester us to make such a visit, but we would not even say, "yes" at the first instance. We would only nod after several such persuasions. Parents and other kin would ask our cousins and friends to make such a programme. But look at the younger boys, they have

no *hanko* (a feeling of restraint out of respect of age mixed with hesitation, modesty and lack of confidence).' Sonji, who sat while listening silently all this time, summed up curtly, 'Where is *hanko* these days? Young men follow their wives as calves follow cows.'

There is also a change in the manner in which visits of the younger son-in-law are organized. First, there is a change in his dress. He rarely ties a *potiyo* (turban) while visiting his in-laws'.[1] Secondly, a marked change has occurred in the rituals and celebrations associated with the visit. In the past his visit used to be an occasion to be celebrated, though on a low key, not only by the immediate household but also by relatives and neighbours. As soon as the son-in-law arrived with his friends and kinsmen, a few neighbours and relatives were sent for. While the men settled down and talked, the women cooked dinner. A few neighbours and relatives joined the guests for dinner. Children were asked to inform relatives and neighbouring women to come for a singing session (*gīt gavāṇo*) in honour of the son-in-law. But, for almost a decade now, these practices are on the decline. As the frequency of the visits has increased, celebrations have waned. Consequently, these visits are becoming an affair restricted to the household. As the emerging privacy is convenient for the son-in-law, his deviance from the cultural precept of modesty can be concealed from public censure.

Another noticeable change, with some influence on the shrinking of birth intervals, is the declining parental authority over married daughters. In recent years, some of the castes are withdrawing their hold over married daughters especially regarding their residence in the natal home. Consequently, parents now rarely insist on their married daughters' prolonged stay in the natal home. Parents now send the married daughter away without much fuss whenever she is summoned by her conjugal household. In the past,

---

[1] *Potiyo* (turban) is consideed a sign both of status and adulthood. It is immodest on the part of a son-in-law to be without it while on a visit to his in-laws. Many remarks were made by the elderly about such immodesty. The comment of Vaddi, an old women is typical: 'None of my sons-in-law came with uncovered head. In our times things were much more decent and respectful. These days the sons-in-law come bare-headed (without *potiyo*) as though they were entering their parents' home and not their *havaro* (in-laws' house).'

a married daugher stayed longer in her parental home during the first five years of marriage. She did not visit her conjugal home for one year after *muklāwo*, while her husband visited her once or twice during that year. She made occasional visits to her conjugal household for the next two years. For another two years or so, the bride stayed for almost the same duration in the two houses, gradually tilting the balance towards prolonged residence in the conjugal home with shortened visits to the parental. But recently, the duration of stay after marriage in the parental home has declined in favour of the conjugal home. This has increased her exposure to conception.

### *Indigenous Techniques of Fertility Control*

The understanding of beliefs and practices supporting prevailing birth intervals would be incomplete without probing into indigenous techniquies regulating them. These techniques are concrete expressions of people's notions of the human body and its physiology. What is significant about these techniques is not their actual efficacy in controlling fertility but the claims associated with them.

As the logic underlying the techniques is derived from prevailing notions, a word about their content would be in order. The understanding of human physiology is based on analogies drawn from agricultural production. A woman's body is equated with a field and a man's semen to a with seed.[2] A woman's impregnation is considered similar to the sowing of a field with *bajri* (millet). (*Bajri*, being the staple crop, is frequently mentioned in such statements.) While employing this analogy, it is said that the crop will grow if seeds are sown, while the field will remain fallow if no seed is sown. In the same vein, it is held that if childbirth is not desired, then the seed need not be sown. The option of not sowing the seed can be realized in two ways: abstinence and withdrawal. Abstinence is believed to be an ideal means to avoid conception. Whereas abstinence is institutionalized and culturally upheld, withdrawal is disapproved normatively and practised

---

[2] Dube (1986) has elaborated on this theme through a symbolic analysis of the terms 'earth' and 'seed'.

unobtrusively. As withdrawal is shrouded in secrecy, very few respondents divulged information about this practice. Only three women and one man reported about it.

> Mehra, a man in the early thirties, confided while his wife sat beside me: 'It is not difficult to practise withdrawal. Both of us take slight care at the right moment and we have no fears of conception. Unlike other contraceptives, it involves no hassles.'
>
> A mother concerned about her daughter's excessive fertility suggested this method for avoiding conception. Her daughter, Parti confided: '*Bajri* grows only when you sow the seed. If the field is ploughed without sowing *bajri* (the seed) nothing will grow. This is the formula my mother gave me. And I immediately understood what she meant. It has worked very well with me for so many years.'
>
> Alpu, who had come to visit her parental home, explained why she never revealed to anyone her practice of the withdrawal technique: 'Women cook up stories and make derogatory remarks. It is best if it remains a secret.'

The practice of withdrawal is not popular as it cannot overcome the barrier of cultural modesty. During the initial years of marriage the young couple feels rather reserved in sharing or discussing with each other their sexual experiences or contraceptive techniques. The question of arriving at a consenesus about a certain technique is obviously ruled out. Even later, when a woman learns of the withdrawal method, she is always shy to talk about it to her husband. Invariably, it takes some time before she can break the ice. With a lot of hesitation, a few young women confided that they could not tell this to their husbands, while a few reported that their husbands approved of the technique. Of them, the majority pointed out the paradoxical behaviour of their husbands who did not object to the technique on the face of it, but never really practised it when required.

Local medicines are also used to curtail fertility. In their usage they do not require joint participation of the spouses. These medicines are popular exclusively among middle-aged women since, as we have seen, they are more desperate than men to avoid conception after acquiring the optimum number of children. Women use medicinal preparations in two conditions. Certain preparations are taken immediately after childbirth, while others during normal days as a preventive to avoid conception.

The local medicines are classified into two main categories, depending upon their supposed properties. They are either sticky or cold. A substance is supposed to be sticky in terms of how it gets glued to certain parts of the body. A cold substance is one that is supposed to neutralize body heat. The sticky substances, such as fenugreek, rice and fuller's earth, are usually taken immediately after childbirth. These are supposed to be effective soon after child delivery, when the woman's body is considered to be tender. These substances are believed to reach the uterus and block entry into the womb before the body regains its original toughness. During the course of such medication, the *huāvaḍ* is postponed to enhance the efficacy of the medicine.

One reason why younger mothers do not use these medicines is that they are under closer observation of elderly women of the household during the first few childbirths. They have no access even to space and time to experiment with such medicines. After having a few children mothers in their middle age become more independent in deciding about and procuring these medicines and the ingredients of their *huāvaḍ*.

Medicines understood to have properties of cooling the body can be taken any time except during the post-partum period (*jāpa*). One of the medicines consists of ground carrot seeds mixed with *hīro* (a sweet prepared with *ghee*, wheat flour, sugar/jaggery and water). It is taken for a few days on an empty stomach soon after the menstrual cycle is over. As soon as the course is over, it is considered mandatory for a woman to consume *lādu* (a sweet) prepared with five kilograms of ghee. The latter course lasts for about a fortnight. People also believe that if the quantity of ghee is less than the specified amount, the woman is likely to become blind. This makes the medicine so expensive that many mothers-in-law do not allow their daughters-in-law to try it.

Certain other cooling medicines are believed to have no adverse effect and can be taken any time other than *jāpa*. These are considered helpful in advancing menopause. Therefore, they are tried mostly by women in their late thirties or early forties. As these medicines are expensive, they are usually taken under the pretext of body ache and sore eyes (a common ailment in desert conditions). It is difficult for poorer women to take these medicines due to their high cost. Many other women are deterred by severe restrictions associated with the medicines. These include avoiding the sun, smoke, strenuous work and extreme weather.

The most secretive and least popular of all birth control methods is abortion. A clear distinction is made between induced abortion and spontaneous abortion or miscarriage. The former is called *tābar pataknọ* or *adūro pataknọ* (to drop a baby on purpose or to drop prematurely) and the latter *adūro paḍno* or *bichate utarṇo* (to fall down prematuely or to slip in between). The distinction indicates whether the abortion is intended or not. Each carries a different implication for both the mother and the expert attendants. Miscarriage is considered an undesirable accident or mishap. It is believed to be a punishment ordained by the divine for some poor karma or sinful act, or inflictions of an evil spirit. On the other hand, induced abortion is a sinful act liable to severe punishment in this or the other life. The general disapproval associated with induced abortion is conveyed through a proverb, '*Sāt pūra ne ēk adūro* (literally, seven normal child deliveries are equal to one abortion).' It is a more agonizing experience for the woman. Acute fear is associated with abortion, both in its physical as well as moral consequences.

As mentioned earlier, the foetus is believed to have a life of its own and is conferred personhood as though it were already born. Aborting a foetus is akin to killing a person. A generous amount of grain for birds and ants, and fodder for cows is distributed as atonement. This is the most common measure adopted to earn *punya*, or to expiate any act considered to be sinful. Even though abortion is severely criticized, a few women have resorted to it in an emergency.

> Meerki, aged 37 and on the verge of becoming a mother-in-law, took several hot *ukāḷis* (infusions) in desperation and terribly upset her system. She had to ultimately approach a *dai* and request her to save her life. After a great deal of persuasion, the *dai* agreed to help. She related the event to me: 'Fortunately for Meerki the abortion did come through. Meerki would have died otherwise. I did it because I was not the principal sinner in the matter. She had already initiated the trouble. I just saved her life. Though I share the lesser *pāp* (religious punishment) for the act, I added an amount equal to the money Meerki paid me and bought grain and fooder as reparation. I didn't earn anythng.'

As mentioned earlier, women likely to become mothers-in-law in about a year's time are particularly careful to avoid conception. They try several methods to stop procreation, but if they happen to conceive, they are usually desperate to get rid of the pregnancy.

Although abortion in general is considered a sin, it is resorted to mostly if a woman conceives either before *muklāwo* or after becoming a mother-in-law. Although the extent of expiation for all abortions is the same, pre-marital pregnancy is not tolerated. Abortions in such cases are closely guarded secrets, though they rarely remain so for long. I could discover one such case:

> Kamma had to undergo an abortion to save her household from disrepute as she had conceived before *muklāwo* (a rare event, as most girls are sent to their conjugal households around puberty).

The local nurse and *dai* are also of the view that abortion as such is a sinful act. To abort is to accumulate bad deeds which are enough to ruin the next incarnation. They did not want to suffer in the next birth. The nurse reasoned that she already had three daughters, believed to be a result of poor karma in the past birth. She feared that doing such sinful acts would mean a worse after-life. She maintained a clean image in the village by not handling such cases. Also, she refused to do abortions to avoid legal complications that could arise on mishandling them.

## *Conclusion*

Contrary to some demographers' assumption that rural people rarely control their fertility, people in Mogra practise fertility control albeit through elaborate customs. Reproduction is not left entirely to the caprices of natural impulses. The fecundity duration is not fully realized in actual behaviour. Fertility is brought to an end much before the end of the fecundity period.

Social norms regulate and control fertility in terms of the developmental phase of the husband-wife couple's fertility career. The norm proscribes procreation after a certain optimum number of surviving children. The woman's interest in the conjugal household and its economy increases with her stay there. With the birth of a few children her status increases, and along with it her role and responsibilities. Her roles get more diversified with the progression of the household. Her status as a mother, the multiple roles associated with it, and the growing role-conflict emanating from the progression of the household, become quite demanding. The birth of an additional child after achieving the socially prescribed optimum number of children further complicates matters. She thus reaches the culmination stage of her fertility career.

Social practices prohibit childbirth after a couple's married children enter their fertility careers. The social norms operate through the organization of nuptial space for spouses, the norm of optimum family size, the regulation of birth intervals, and the culmination phase in the developmental process of the couple's fertility carreer. In addition, indigenous techniques are adopted to supplement the observance of these norms. Among them are abstinence, attempts to advance menopause, and folk medication.

The social institutions and indigenous practices of fertility control are woven symbolically into values and beliefs related to the fertility career. These are not blind to the health of both the mother and the child. The observance of various abstinences and other practices to avoid conception provide sufficient time for the mother to recuperate. Some of the fertility control practices are even rooted in human physiology, as for instance, liberal breast-feeding to delay ovulation.

CHAPTER 7

# Modern Fertility Control: People's Experiences

Modern means of fertility control have made inroads into Mogra in recent times. Since these means were intorduced mainly under the national Family Planning Programme (FPP), this chapter focusses on people's response to it. How did FPP find its way into the village? What do people think about it? Do they evaluate its philosophy and techniques and then accept/reject the total package, or do they judiciously select certain components? Does FPP reinforce prevailing fertility practices or interfere with them? How is it seen in relation to indigenous practices of fertility control discussed in Chapter 6? How do these varying frameworks coexist in the village? What is the process of acceptance of FPP in the context of prevailing norms, values and cosmology of fertility and its control?

Although India is the first country in the world to have officially introduced FPP in 1952 along with the five year plans, the people of Mogra became familiar with it during the national emergency of 1975–7. A state of national emergency was declared in June 1975 family planning then entered the forefront of Indian politics. The family planning compaign during this period was more intense than at any other time in India, using sometimes coercive methods for its acceptance. During the 22-month period 11 million people (many of them unmarried, many overage, and many with less than two children) were sterilized compared with 1.3 million in the preceding year (see Bose 1988: 50–55 for a detailed account).

Despite its official introduction in 1952, FPP took an unusually long time to reach Mogra like many other villages in the country. FPP evaluation studies and KAP surveys reveal the poor penetraton of FPP in the country, especially in rural areas. Although the people of Mogra had heard about the birth control programme and techniques propagated by the government before 1975–7, they had little clarity about it. The spread of FPP in rural India began with an emphasis on sterilization through the 'camp approach' in the early seventies, especially in Kerala and Gujarat.

FPP embodies a set of assumptions ubiquitous in most family planning packages in developing countries. Three of them need special mention. First, there is a general Neo-Malthusian and western view that increasing population means a constant drain of the limited resources of the nation and that fertility control is a necessary step without which economic development would be retarded. The second assumption, also borrowed from western experience, is that fertility behaviour is based on the decision and planning of the individual couple. The third assumption is that the couple do not feel the need to plan the family due to their ignorance of the effective use of contraceptives, and the importance of spacing children for the health of both mother and child. Effective fertility control is, therefore, possible only by adequately motivating and enlightening the couple to practice family planning.

As we have seen, people in Mogra subscribe to a complex set of practices and beliefs about fertility, spacing of births, mother and child health, and optimum family size. But FPP reflects little knowledge of people's reproductive beliefs and practices and is actually at variance with them. Therefore, people's response to FPP has been neither passive nor ignorant. In other words, they have been assessing the package and comparing it with their own practices of fertility behaviour.

The norms, values, social practices and related cosmology discussed in Chapter 6 are too complex to permit an uncritical acceptance of FPP in its totality. As discussed in Chapter 4, there exists in Mogra a complex institutional arrangement to take overall care of the mother's and child's physical and emotional health. The prevailing beliefs, rituals and folk medicines play a vital role in this regard. The prevailing practices take care of the parturient mother's recovery. A person who does not suffer from a serious ailment is considered to be helathy.[1]

The data in this chapter pertains to people's knowledge of FPP, their experiences of its practice, and evaluation of some of its popular components. the information was obtained from ever married men as well as women in Mogra during prolonged interviews. Owing to people's secretive attitude towards most contraceptive measures, data collection regarding FPP relied largely on unstructured interviews and group discussions. Clues about people using modern contraceptives came from their close friends and relatives. However, it was not easy to extract information about use of modern contractives. Hanging on with people who were said to have some experience of modern contraceptives did yield data occasionally. But information on sterilization was rarely a secret. Questions about sterilization, the technique, place where sterilized, etc. were included in the interview schedule itself. Unstructured interviews were used for obtaining additional information about men and women who had opted for sterilization.

### *Some Experiences with FPP*

To most people in Mogra, FPP is synonymous with terminaton of fertility, i.e., sterilization. Such a perception is typical of the trend prevalent in most developing societies, particularly in the Asian region (U. N. 1981). Even when some persons have a vague knowledge about certain contraceptives, they seldom use them regularly. Both contraceptives and sterilization are seen by the people as governmental means to curtail or stop childbirth (locally called, *baccha band karṇo*; literally, stop the children) contraceptives that cause inconvenience or embarrassment are discarded. The inconvenience and/or embarrassment is not entirely without justification.

Kamala, aged 35, mother of six children, said about her experience

---

[1] People's notion of health is indicated commonly through two words, fat (*māto*) and thin (*thākoḍo*), meaning good and poor health respectively. A bodily disorder impeding normal course of life is categorized as illness. If an ailment does not hamper one's daily routine, the person is rarely considered as being seriously ill.

> of the condoms: 'They (condoms) are a menace. It is always difficult to keep them from the reach of children. No corner or niche in the house remains hidden from them. They are always on the look out for something to eat or play with. A condom is like a balloon for them. What an embarrassing sight it is when the condom is blown and people laugh meaningfully!'
>
> Mangli Sargara, mother of three children, disclosed her experience of the condom: 'Disposing of it is always a problem. There scarcely is a moment when you can bury it without being seen.'
>
> Paani, a young Patel mother with four children, had her own experience of the condom: 'One can't carry it all the time What if one needs it in the field?'
>
> Sugan reported about Mohni's agonizing experience of IUD: 'Ever since the insertion, her menstrual cycle was disrupted. She bled incessantly for three months and turned pale. She ultimately had to get it removed, or she would have died leaving behind her children to ruin.'
>
> Alpu had once experimented with contraceptive oral pills. she reported: 'I would always forgot its schedule. For me it never worked.'

In people's experinece contracptives threaten whatever little privacy they have (insufficient in any case by urban middle class standards). To handle contraceptives is to risk public disapproval or ridicule. The contraceptives also intrude into people's definition of item and freedom. In the case of pills it is extremely difficult for a woman to maintain a specific time schedule. Condoms are a perpetual source of embarrassment for both husband and wife. They restrict freedom of sex outside the house—in the fields or any other hideout. Disposing of them is not easy either. They are not easily perishable, and consequently have to be buried carefully to avoid children playing with them.

The natue of housing in Mogra is unlike urban apartments or bungalows. The notion of a room in Mogra is different from its dictionary meaning. It ranges from a proper enclosed structure with a ceiling, a floor and a door, to a straw shed with walls on three, and sometimes only two, sides. Each house has at least one proper room to store valuables, clothes, etc, locally called *ori*. Although houses in Mogra are quite spacious, construction is sparse. Many houses do not have a separate kitchen. An average house has about three rooms (including sheds). In addition, there are cattle sheds.

All household members have an almost equal claim and access to rooms in the house. The store room (*ori*) is accessible to all household members. It is mostly locked. But when opened children are curious to know why. It is not easy to escape children's vigil and take the contraceptives away. It is not easy to clench the shelved. The sense of individual privacy is discouraged. It is rare for a person to have a room exclusively to oneself. No couple in Mogra has a bedroom to itself all day and night. The newly married couple have a separate room exclusively to themselves only at night. In about two years of marriage, the couple begins to use a shed or such other site away from the courtyard where most of the household members sleep at night. Sleeping arrangements have been discussed in the previous chapter. A near lack of privacy during day time and the sleeping arrangement at night are hardly conductive to regular use of contraceptives. The problem is more acute in larger and complex households, where the early years of one's marriage are spent. Later one's own children share the rooms and other space, allowing little privacy to a couple.

The experience of using modern contraceptives is seldom bereft of inconvenience or other problems. Whereas couples try contraception with a desire to stop fertility, their actual use confronts them with a series of pain and discomfort, besides failing frequently in curtailing fertility. People disapprove and discontinue the use of modern contraceptives and prefer an alternative devoid of problems and perils. They believe that there exists a more simple and convenient contraceptive in the form of an injection, which is not available to them partly due to its exorbitant cost and partly due to the ignorance of most doctors and medical personnel about its very existence. Three women past their child bearing age claimed to have administerd such injections on themselves. One of them related her experience regarding what she considered was an injectable contraceptive.

> Jamni, an old Patel woman who had two sons and five daughters, confided in me: 'I, along with two of my friends, had taken a contraceptive injection as all of us had enough children. The injection was effective as none of us had any child after that. And in five years time we reached menopause. Unfortunately the chemist who administered the injection is dead. He would have been so

> helpful if he were alive today. He could have rescued several women desiring that injection.'

Other women also believed strongly in the existence of an injectable conveptive. For instance:

> Haski Suthar, mother of five, always complained against me for not arranging her the most sought after injection that prevents conception for a duration of five years. She said: 'All these (available contraceptives) are useless. We can't handle them. But an injection would be so good. It would only pain little when pricked. And then one need not bother about anything (typical problems associated with the use of prevailing contraceptives)'.

Several similar comments were made by many other women desiring such an injection, although local doctors seldom confirmed their views. Despite popular belief regarding the existence of a contraceptive injection, I was unable to gather more data. Therefore, I cannot say much about it.

Sterilization is another method tried in Mogra. It was introduced during the national emergency by school teachers, doctors, nurses and other officials visiting the village occasionally. Official propaganda and urban contact also exposed people to this new idea. A few of these officials persuaded people to sterilize themselves. They exerted pressure on people in order to fulfill their target of sterilizations. All sterilizations except one were performed on men in camps in a neighbouring village during the emergency. Nevertheless, sterilization was strongly disapproved. People were critical of it. To them it was a matter of shame and thus unwelcome. At the level of cosmology, it was a sinful act. On the other hand, tubectomy was believed to interfere with a woman's physical capability for hard agricultural work, be it back-breaking tasks or the transporting of heavy loads on head.

Most of these notions continue to hold good in Mogra (see Caldwell *et al* 1984: 201 for an account of such skepticism in Karnataka). The post-operative complications are feared to incapacitate people and bring a couple's sexual life to a virtual end. These apprehensions were strengthened by the initial sterilization experiences of people during the emergency. These experiences are still alive in the collective memory of the people. They construct their images, meanings and opinions from the details of these cases. Often the experiences of the sterilized reinforce people's fears and strengthen their views against it. It becomes a common body of knowledge for people, especially when it results in some complication. The news spreads like wild fire through word of mouth, recurs in gossip, and becomes common knowledge in the village.

> Meeri, mother of two sons and a daughter, the first and the only woman in Mogra, to be sterilized during the emergency suffered from numerous complications soon after the operation. Her physical ailment, depression and inability to work hard led to terrible disapproval and criticism in the household. She had continuous body ache and severe backache. To top it all, the household elders criticized her because she could not work as hard as her sisters-in-law (husband's brothers wives). Rather than being sympathized for remaining unwell she was rebuked and blamed for being a work shirker. The whole experience was agonizing till she separated from the complex household and her growing children actively assisted her in the household work. Meeri's experience became a strong deterrent for other women against sterilization.
>
> Saori, a Harijan woman had a son a few years after her husband was sterilized during the emergency. Although technically the operation had failed, the ridicule continued to be hurled at the household and the couple for several months. Even till a few years later a reference to her made people exchange meaningful gestures or some derogatorey comment. Only when laparoscopy[2] failed in two female cases did people accept the possibility of the failure of sterilization.

Such discouraging encounters are part of the meaning assigned to sterilization. These meanings, as part of collective memory, contribute in dissuading other people from accepting it. The fear of prolonged post-surgical weakness and pain encourage few people to opt for it even when social norms expect them to stop procreation. As modern means of fertility control are not incommon use, any post-surgical complication is given scarce attention. It is also clear to these women that they cannot seek any concessions in household or other work on this ground. The

---

[2] Laparoscopy is considered to be an operaton conducted with the help of *beejḷi* and *doorveeṇ*, literally, electricity and telescope.

seven cases of sterilization during 1975–7 acted as negative references for others in Mogra. The post-operative complications and the consequent miserable condition of Meeri deterred women from sterilizing themselves.

As the new technique of laparoscopy has fewer complications, several younger mothers have opted for it. Each time a few women get sterilized by this technique in a camp, others are curious to know if there are any adverse after-effects. When a woman does not suffer from any, one or two of her friends and relatives (who have achieved the socially optimum number of children) begin to contemplate sterilizing themselves. For about seven years after the emergency no one in Mogra opted for sterilization.

But things have not remained the same. By 1982–3 there emerged a new trend among women to volunteer for sterilization. Birth control (laparoscopy) camps in Mogra and its vicinity had become active during the early eighties. The more convenient alternative of laparoscopy with few complications was an added attraction. It was during this period that female sterilizations outnumbered male ones.

> Sangari, a widow in her early fifties, confided in me that female sterilization is safer these days: 'The problem of security is mounting, and it is not safe for a solitary woman to go to the fields. Men's morals are fast degenerating. In such a condition it is safer for a woman to get sterilized so that if an accident (rape) happens she is safe. If her husband is vasectomized she would be ruined.'

Laparoscopy is becoming popular among a small minority of women. They find it convenient as well as less demanding on their schedule. It is perceived to be different from the usual notion of surgery. 'It involves only a prick,' is the usual comment. Thus, the numerous fears associated with a surgical operation (particularly tubectomy and vasectomy) are substantially contained. Laparoscopy is gaining popularity over tubectomy also because it does not require abstaining from heavy work and sexual life for long. There is little fear of serious incapacitation as compared to other methods of sterilization. It does not upset the daily round of women's activities. Little forethought is required. A casual slip out of the house, akin to a brief gossip session or a siesta, is all that is required. In real terms, women have to abstain from home for only an hour or two. It is possible for them to walk back home on their own within half an hour of the laparoscopy 'prick'. None of the women in Mogra experienced any difficulty in resuming or supervising work after they returned home. All this is in sharp contrast to tubectomy which requires considerable planning, including leaving the domestic scene for a few days.

### *Acceptance of Sterilization: Modern Techniques in a Traditional Context*

Although I have clarified in Chapter 1 how tense has been used, it is necessary to reiterate it. While the discussion of sterilizations till they were done is in the past tense, the discussion of modern means of fertility control in the post-sterilization period is in the present tense. Of course, other general observations are also made in the present tense.

As already mentioned, my probe into fertility experiences of 713 ever married women and some of their husbands included questions on fertility control, especially through sterilization. In all, 64 persons (45 women and 19 men) were sterilized between 1975 and 1985 (when the present fieldwork was done). To gather additional data relating to sterilization, I had especially long probing sessions with most of the sterilized women and a few men.

As discussed in Chapter 6, fertility behaviour in Mogra is far from being unrestrained and unregulated. Fertility follows a certain trajectory, a certain span of reproductive career in a couple's life. The fertility career is marked by a socially prescribed beginning and an end. It is controlled through the prevailing institutions, norms, the associated statuses and roles. It may appear that acceptance of sterilization by a couple points to a radical change in their attitude to family size. But my inquiry reveals that they have all followed the basic norm of fertility. Their notions of the optimum number of children in the family have altered little. There exists a contradiction between the expectations that planners and people have of sterilization. This contradiction may be explained through an analysis of fertility behaviour of persons who accepted sterilization.

The 64 persons constitute nearly 9% of the total number of 713 ever married women or their husbands in Mogra. Their sex distribution (45 women and 19 men) follows the larger Indian pattern, namely, more women than men have undergone sterilization (Mahadevan and Sumangala 1987: 130 report this for India in genral and for Andhra pradesh and Kerala in particular). Of the 45 sterilized women, 17 accepted tubectomy and 28 laparoscopy.

Of the 64 sterilized persons, 60 were sterilized before the age of 40, and only four after. Most of them belonged to the age range of 26 to 40. Even within this range the majority were between 26 and 35 years. These figures show that the need for sterilization after 40 is not felt so acutely. The main reason is that indigenous methods (primarily abstinence) are adopted to put an end to one's fertility career after this age. This is also the stage when the fecundity of older women is coming to an end.

Proportionately more men engaged in the relatively modern occupations of business and government service have got themselves sterilized than those in the traditional occupations of animal husbandry, agriculture, artisanship, and wage labour. Also, more men in business and service have vasectomized themselves as compared to their wives. This may be explained by the fact that sterilization is considered to be debilitating and therfore inhibitive of hard physical labour. Because these men perform less strenous tasks than their wives they preferred to get themselves sterilized. Their wives do more strenuous jobs because they continue to engage in agriculture. If they were to get sterilized, the enitre household economy based on agriculture would suffer. Of the 19 vasectomies, seven were performed during the emergency period of 1975–7, under severe pressure and threat. Most of the rest were accepted by men who either live in urban areas and/or employed in urban centres. The influence of urban ethos has some role to play in their case.

The place of sterilization is important to show the extent of motivation, courage, and social approval that the concerned individual has. Those more determined to sterilize are less fearful of surgery, have greater approval of their act from other members of the household, and usually get themselves sterilized in hospitals in the nearby city. Of the 64 cases, 20 got themselves sterilized in hospitals, a few of them primarily because they were predominantly urban-based. The remaining 44 were sterilized in various camps organized in the village or its vicinity. Eight of them were sterilized by coercion during the emergency.

The feeling of security is stronger in a sterilization camp by virtue of its proximity to one's home. The fear of surgery in a hospital has resulted in a larger number of sterilizations in camps. In some cases of laparoscopy, women have dared to take the step without a clear consensus or approval of their household members. One of the reasons for their courage is the understandng that laparoscopy in Mogra and its vicinity is more convenient than tubectomy in many ways.

Survival of a few children, including sons, is a crucial factor behind the decission to sterilize. All the sterilized persons have as many children as the non-sterilized. Their average number of childbirths, child mortality and child survival are not very different from those of the others. The average fertility of the sterilized is 5.68 children per couple (husband and wife), while the average child mortality is one child per couple at the time of sterilization. Each of the sterilized persons had on an average about five surviving children, with nearly three surviving sons, out of six children born to them. Only six couples had one surviving son each, while 25 had two; 16 had three; and 12 had four sons each at the time of the wife's/husband's sterilization. As already noted, to have only one son is to put the parents in a dangerously precarious condition.

Most of the sterilized husbands/wives having only one son had sterilized themselves after having several daughter, and after having reconciled with their fate (of having only one son). More than one half of the sterilized (36 out of 64) have experienced no child loss in their fertility careers. Table 7.1 depicts fathers/mothers by number of children born, dead, and surviving to them at the time of sterilization. Of the 64 persons, 28 have experienced the agony of the death of one or more children. Eight of them lost one child, 11 lost two, three lost as many, four persons lost four and two lost five or more children each. But none got sterilized before assuring themselves of the survival of the required number of children. Forty two of the 64 have 4–6 children surviving, 15 have 1–3, 6 have 7–9, and one has more than nine surviving children. The sex break-up worked out from Table 7.1 shows that

TABLE 7.1 *Distribution of fathers/mothers by children born, dead and surviving at the time of sterilization*

| *No. of Chld* | *Number of fathers/mothers with* | | | | | | | | |
|---|---|---|---|---|---|---|---|---|---|
| | *Children born* | | | *Children dead* | | | *Children surviving* | | |
| | *S* | *D* | *T* | *S* | *D* | *T* | *S* | *D* | *T* |
| 0 | 0 | 3 | 0 | 49 | 40 | 36 | 0 | 3 | 0 |
| 1 | 5 | 16 | 0 | 8 | 14 | 8 | 6 | 21 | 0 |
| 2 | 23 | 15 | 2 | 3 | 7 | 11 | 25 | 21 | 3 |
| 3 | 11 | 9 | 11 | 3 | 2 | 3 | 16 | 10 | 12 |
| 4 | 12 | 12 | 10 | 1 | 0 | 4 | 12 | 3 | 14 |
| 5+ | 13 | 9 | 41 | 0 | 1 | 2 | 5 | 6 | 35 |

Note: chld= children; S= Sons; D= Daughters; T= Total.

more sons (178) than daughters (137) were surviving in the case of a majority of parents when they sterilized themselves. Thirty eight of them had proportionately more sons and 10 more daughters surviving. Only 12 had an equal number of sons and daughters. The value of sons is indicated by the fact that three persons got themselves sterilized without any daughter being born to them, while none got sterilized without the birth of a son or soon after the birth of daughters.

The sex proportion of a couple's children dead before the time of sterilization is important to place it in perspective. While only 15 sterilized persons had experienced a son's death, as many as 24 had lost their daughters, and 36 had lost none. It is well-known that sex distribution of children at birth is in favour of boys all over the world. So also, of 315 children born to 64 persons, 178 (56.5%) were boys and 137 (43.5%) girls. The data on child mortality for all 713 couples in Mogra discussed in Chapter 5 reveals higher female mortality. In the case of 64 couples, the survival rate among boys is almost 85% compared to 72% among girls. Male child mortality (15.16%) is lower than that of females (28.46%).

But these averages should not convey that every couple had experienced child mortality. Although 36 persons did not suffer directly the tribulations of child mortality, they had indirectly experienced it occurring around them. Thus, they did not want to take any risk, and got themselves sterilized only after having at least two surviving sons and a daughter, normatively held to be the minimum. No one decided on sterilization before a few of their children's survival could be hoped for. This criterion also applies to the youngest age group (up to 25 years) of the sterilized persons. All the children born to them were surviving at the time of sterilization. On an average, the younger couples had nearly four children each before one of the spouses got sterilized, because they did not find it worthwhile to continue to bear more children. Child death after one's sterilization cannot be ruled out. Of the 64 sterilized persons, four lost one son, and three lost one daughter each after their sterilization. The fear of the possibility of child mortality after sterilization rarely encourages couples to get themselves sterilized as soon as they have two or three children, including one or two sons. There is only one couple with two sons, three couples with two sons and one daughter each, and two couples with one son and two daughters each who put a stop to their reproduction by means of sterilization. None of these six couples lost any child.

The data shows a marked decrease in child mortality in recent times, especially during the past decade as mentioned in Chapters 3 and 5. Persons belonging to different ages have different experiences of child mortality. The younger perosons have lost fewer children than did the older ones. Mothers above the age of 30 have lost 22–25% of the children born to them, those in the age group of 26 to 30 have lost 11% of the children born, and those below 25 have lost none. The general experience of child survival in the community assured these young persons of the survival of their children after they had over two sons and a daughter on an average.

A comparison of the average number of child births and child deaths per person (see Table 7.2) shows that people get themselves sterilized only after assuring the survival of the socially expected number of children. Persons who did not lose any child were the only ones to have sterilized themselves at a very early age. Those persons who suffered higher mortality of children sterilized at a sulater age. Child mortality dissuades couples from accepting sterilization. Couples as well as their relatives wish to see that at least a few children survive. To ensure about five surviving children, including at least two sons, it is thought rational to have

TABLE 7.2 *Distribution of average fertility, child mortality and child survival per couple by mother's age*

| *Mother's age (in years)* | *Fertility* | *Child mortality* | | | *Child survival* |
|---|---|---|---|---|---|
| | | *Before sterilizing* | *After sterilizing* | *Total* | |
| 21–25 | 3.6 | | 0.07 | 0.07 | 3.5 |
| 26–30 | 5.0 | 0.7 | — | 0.7 | 4.3 |
| 31–35 | 6.2 | 1.3 | 0.2 | 1.5 | 4.7 |
| 36–40 | 8.0 | 1.3 | 0.5 | 1.8 | 6.2 |
| 41–45 | 8.0 | 1.8 | 0.2 | 2.0 | 6.0 |
| 46+ | 7.0 | 3.0 | | 3.0 | 4.0 |

one or two extra children. This logic is used even by those parents who have not lost any children. The termination of reproductivity is thus pushed somewhat further and the time range of active fertility is stretched. The total number of children born thus increases as parents keep a margin for losses. Table 7.2 shows how fertility and child loss are concomitant with delayed birth control among the sterilized. Older mothers have higher average fertility as well as child mortality, compared to younger mothers. But the average child survival figures show lesser variation across age groups (3.5 for mothers aged between 21 and 25, and four for those above 46).

The distribution of fertility and mortality by mother's age is an important indication that a person does not decide to get sterilized exclusively on the basis of his/her own fertility experiences. The couple do not view their fertility experiences in isolation from those of others around them before deciding to stop procreation. Of the 64 persons who terminated their fertility career, senior mothers aged 36 and above had higher fertility as well as child mortality, in contrast to mothers in the 21 to 35 age group. This can be explained by the collective experience of mortality being an important aspect of a couple's behavior as discussed in Chapter 5. Even if an individual could escape the trauma of child mortality, the couple continue to be influenced by the wider experience of child mortality in the community. As a corollary, it is rare to find a person sterilizing him/herself after one son and one daughter, or two sons and one daughter, are born. He/she waits for a few years to be assured of child survival before putting a stop to procreation.

However, with the recent decline in child deaths in the community, younger couples have had realtively lesser exposure as well as self-experience of child mortality. They have lesser fear of losing their children than their seniors. They feel little need to produce more children to compensate for an eventual loss, while older parents with greater exposure to child mortality sterilize only after sufficiently providing for the loss of a few children. But this does not mean that they go on producing children as long as they can. The distribution in Table 7.2, especially of child survival, supports this observation.

Another important factor for sterilization is attainment of the status of mother-in-law. Of the sterilized women, 16 are aged 36 and above—an age when most women are likely to become mothers-in-law. Of the 16 women, as many as 14 had become so before sterilization. One mother-in-law got herself sterilized even though she was below 35. Several young women aged between 31 and 35 also got themselves sterilized as they were to become mothers-in-law in the coming one or two years.

The mothers-in-law perfer to end their fertility to avoid conception and consequent ridicule. In addition, they have the advantage of grown up daughters or daughters-in-law living with them whose presence is helpful in overcoming any ill-effects of sterilization. They take up major household responsibilities and enable the sterilized woman to have the required rest.

Thus, sterilization remains within the traditional value-frame for older as well younger couples. It helps stop childbirths after one's grown-up children enter their reproductive life. On the other hand, sterilization enables the couple to avoid the birth of an unwanted child. This is particularly so when the couple has secured the socially optimum fertility and child survival. Sterilization is adopted by one of the spouses as a means to an end, once they fulfill the conventional fertility norm.

The limited scope and relevance of FPP in Mogra may be compared with Kara and Sinha's (1987) study of the impact of FPP in India in general and Orissa in particular. Their study points out that FPP made little dent, as the number of living children in all cases of tubectomy and vasectomy exceeded three. There is sufficient empirical evidence that people observe strictly the social norms of fertility behavior. The Khanna villagers (Wyon and Gordon 1971) accepted contraceptives only as far as they dovetailed with the norms. Contraception did not alter the community norm as to when to have children, how many to have, and when to stop having them. Only women who were over 30 and approaching the traditional terminal stage of child bearing used contraceptive tablets. Instead of cutting down the birth rate, the tablets enabled them to live up to traditional norms with more modern techniques. Similarly, Dandekar (1959) observes that the attitude towards family planning was more favourable among couples with three to five children in the six rural communities she studied in India. FPP could only narrow the gap between the socially expected and the actual family size. It reinforces traditional ideas of family size and fertility by shortening the active fertility duration.

Our material suggests that the people who adopted sterilization have in no way digressed from existing norms about the socially optimum family size. The family planning package is accepted only to the extent that it is instrumental in supporting expected fertility behaviour. Although the technique of sterilization to control fertility is unconventional and its adoption a sort of deviation, it hardly upsets prevailing meanings and practices associated with the traditional reproductive career. Similarly, sterilization, especially by laparoscopy, does not interfere with a woman's routine activities. Although people do not deviate from their cosmologies in accepting sterilization as a technique to terminate fertility, they are rather indifferent to the meanings associated with FPP by planners. This is the context in which FPP is locally unpackaged.

A few of the 68 educated and *naukri*-(salaried job) holding fathers in Mogra are not identical with their illiterate counterparts in fertility behaviour. The former do adopt some modern birth control techniques but only after achieving the socially expected minimum, i.e. at least two sons and a daughter.

Kana Patel is a college drop-out and clerk in a government

department. He has three children with over four years of interval between each of them. His eldest child, a daughter, is married. His wife got herself sterilized a year before their daughter's *muklāwo*.
Anil Charan, with a Ph.D. degree, has nearly five years' gap between his two sons.
Shera Patel, employed in defence services, has three years' interval between each of his six children.
Inda, a young childless Raika, employed as a police constable, feels awkward that his mother is pregnant, although he has been married for two years.
Binja Patel, a school teacher in his late twenties, has stopped bearing further children after having three of them (two sons and a daughter).
Gokal Bhambi, a school teacher, put an end to procreation after having four children (three sons and a daughter).

The above examples enable us to discern that education and *naukri* together make a mark at least on some couples' fertility behaviour but only insofar as they adopt modern measures of control after they achieve the socially minimum fertility. However, in the case of several other couples, this combination has little influence on their fertility.

Shera Patel sent his wife for tubectomy when his three sons and two daughters, of the six children born, were surviving with good health. He allowed tubectomy primarily because of the compulsions of urban ethos, to avoid being ridiculed for having a large number of children, or feeling awkward in social gatherings where his counterparts have fewer children. Even his illiterate counterparts in the village do not consider it proper to have more children after these many.

Inda felt awkward to see his mother pregnant more because of the traditional norm that enjoins termination of fertility when the offsprintg are married.

Other educated *naukri*-holders tend to follow traditional fertility norms more closely.

Despite education and urban jobs, Ajay, a Charan clerk and father of three, Hetu, a Charan peon and father of six daughters, and Kewal, a Patel factory worker with two children, have two years' spacing each between their children, which is in conformity with what others follow in the village. The only Charan girl, Ansu, is married to a lawyer in another town and holds an M.Sc. degree.

> She has had five daughters in 10 years of marriage. She will not stop conceiving till she has a son.

Irrespective of urban jobs or the level of education, social expectations and values regarding sex and number of surviving children continue to dominate a couple's decision to stop or continue child bearing. The individual couple rarely decide their fertility career independent of social norms and compulsions from kin, neighbours and the community. This is clear from the number of children born to educated and *naukri*-holding parent(s).

### *Decision to get Sterilized*

Despite the non-interference of FPP with prevailing fertility norms, sterilization is not unanimously approved. As its practice is unconventional, it evokes disparaging remarks, ranging from opprobrium to ridicule from people. Nevertheless, sterilization occupies a place within the permissible range of deviance.

Almost every woman in Mogra is in a dilemma while deciding about sterilization. A number of countervailing factors impede her decision. First of all it interferes with hard labour and what is worse she can secure no exemption from household chores on this count. Secondly, dependence on senior members of the household makes it mandatory for her to take their permission. In this respect, men are more independent and can take their own decision without seeking the concurrence of their wives or senior household members.

Women consider many factors before they opt for sterilization. We have already discussed the desire of mothers with growing children to terminate their fertility career. Also, a couple's fertility is terminated only when they have attained the eligibility to do it. This does not mean that the eligibility to stop procreation leads automatically to a decision to get sterilized. Sterilization is not accepted as though it were a normative precept or an undisputed maxim. Quite the contrary. Both men and women encounter moments of wavering before making up their mind. Women are of course free to ventilate their agony, but they do not enjoy the same freedom as men do to get sterilized.

Even if a woman is keen, she has to consider the reactions of her husband and other close relatives, especially those in the conjugal household. At the same time she has her own fears about surgery and its adverse after-effects, which in popular opinion renders people incapacitated. As regards vasectomy, people believe that, 'male operation is like castrating a calf. A sterilized male cannot be a bull.' Similarly, there are apprehensions that sterilized women will suffer pain in the limbs, including backache and other ailments that reduce stamina.

A person is initially confronted with all popular fears, in the process of deciding to sterilize. During this phase, the fears are sorted out individually. Not all women manage to overcome the apprehensions and remain indecisive. A few men and women confessed to me that they were scared of surgery, and dropped the idea of getting sterilized.

Almost all sterilized persons had shared their fears with close friends and relatives. In such informal discussions, the decision is discussed threadbare with a mixture of humour and seriousness. The pros and cons are weighed. While some fears are dispelled, others are reinforced. However, a favourable disposition resulting from prolonged discussions does not always lead to a positive decision. The discussions that took place in a circle of close friends now shift to the spouses. The spouse with higher motivation to get sterilized takes the initiative. The themes related to sterilization are repeated. In a sense, the state of indecision is prolonged. From the pool of collective memory, the couple recall and discuss other couples' varied experiences. For instance, they recall cases of those who had no post-surgical problems. Those with many children and very little land, those who sterilized soon after having the socially minimum number of children etc., are recalled. During such discussions the spouses waver between the two positions: one, in favouring and the other against. It is rare for husbands to give unqualified permission to their wives for sterilization, especially if they are living in a joint household. In the latter case, parents have greater authority over the couple in such a matter. However, there are also instances where parents are overruled. While the majority of women seek their household elders' permission, most men do not wait for it.

For a woman the permission of the parents-in-law, particularly the mother-in-law, is crucial, if she is residing with them. As a manager of household affairs, the mother-in-law's opinion and judgement matters considerably. As knowledge about post-surgery complications is common, the mother-in-law is apprehensive. She feels concerned primarily about the adverse impact of sterilization on the daughter-in-law's health and hence on the household routine. Her main anxiety is that if the dauther-in-law's health were impaired the household routine would be seriously disrupted. The breakdown would not only burden household resources but also strain its relationships. The common reaction of most mothers-in-law is one of disapproval, reflected in loss of temper. They vent their premonition that the household would be ruined if the daughter-in-law gets sterilized.

These initial reactions are usually followed by more definite responses. They are of three types. First, the mother-in-law might leave the entire matter to the son and his wife. While keeping her fingers crossed, she restrains herself to merely explaining the undesirable consequences. In a sense, there is in this posture a conscious attempt to relinquish responsibility in the matter and to shift it on to the couple. This response is indicative of helplessness, an apprehension of the possibility that her words might be dishonoured. This kind of response is uncommon, as we shall soon see.

A second typical reaction is outright displeasure. It is justified on the ground that the daughter-in-law's decision is an expression of both ignorance and irresponsibility. It is ignorance insofar as she displays little awareness of the adverse consequences of sterilization on her health and strength to perform hard manual labour. The desire to get sterilized lacks maturity in that it fails to appreciate the problems it is likely to engender. The daughter-in-law is considered irresponsible insofar as her desire ignores the possible breakdown of the household in case of post-surgical complications. The mother-in-law usually resorts to a personal threat by declaring that she would be least responsible in case of any problem. It implies that the daughter-in-law shall have no claim to any concession in work for rest, recuperation and treatment in case sterilization indisposes her.

> Bhoori had pointed out categorically to both of her daughters-in-law who had made up their mind to get sterilized: 'You will have to suffer for your deeds. Don't expect that you will be relieved

> from household work after the operation. You are doing this while knowing fully well how it disables a woman for hard work. You will have to bear the consequences if the household suffers.'

Mothers-in-law thus make it clear that there is little reason to allow the household to suffer by relieving its active members. In such a situation, the husband either chooses to remain silent or wavers between the stands taken by his mother and wife.

> Vena, father of two sons and two daughters, initially agreed to his wife getting sterilized but revoked his concurrence immediately after his mother stressed her disapproval. He had almost agreed with his wife after she convinced him but chose to remain silent when his mother spoke against the decision.

Both the husband and the mother-in-law share a premonition regarding the woman's well-being and its consequent impact on the household. Of course, if they are party to the decision, they would be obliged to allow concessions and bear the added burden.

There is an additional dimension that prevents the mother-in-law from granting direct permission for sterilization. This relates to her managerial shrewdness, which tells her that even if there is no post-surgical complication the daughter-in-law might demand exemption on this count. Therefore, even if the mother-in-law is convinced about the merits of sterilization, it is seldom expressed in her readiness to allow her daughter-in-law to get sterilized. In such a condition the daughter-in-law's decision to get sterilized always appears contrary to the household elders' wishes.

A third typical reaction of the mother-in-law is outright rejection of the very idea of sterilization. They maintain an aggressive posture which unequivocally dismisses the artificial termination of fertility. Most of such mothers-in-law have experienced mortality either of their own children or of their siblings.

> Vaddi, aged 60, experienced the agony of mortality right from her childhood. As a child, she witnessed the loss of a few siblings and as a mother she lost all four children. Such a trail of misfortune continued even in the case of her near relatives, particularly her husband's brother's family (all except one boy and a girl died). Given this background of personal tragedy, Vaddi turned hysterical whenever sterilization was discussed.
>
> Vaddi's adopted son's (her husband's brother's orphaned son's) wife, a mother of four daughters and two sons, recalled vividly: 'I

> wished to get sterilized after I had four children. Upon hearing this *Maaji* (mother-in-law) got so wild that I dared not mention it again. She called insulting names to those who had sterilized. To her they were blind and crazy. How can I tell her that even I want to get sterilized?'

Only a minority of mothers-in-law are disposed favourably. Such a mother-in-law will readily allow her daugher-in-law to go for sterilization. The permission however, derives its rationale not from FPP but from the compulsions of household routine and traditional fertility norms. The household may not depend entirely on the daughter-in-law's labour, because there are grown up children and other household members who can shoulder extra responsibility in an eventuality. Another reason for ready permission may be that the daughter-in-law would have transgressed social norms of fertility by producing more children. Some of her children may have reached marriageable age while others may have embarked upon their fertility careers. Sterilization is thus readily accepted to avoid the ridicule of producing children while one's grandchildren are due.

> Devi, an elderly mother-in-law, is one of the rare examples. She accompanied her daughter-in-law all the way to the city for sterilization. After Devi's eldest granddaughter had been married off to her conjugal home, Devi had a strong desire that her daughter-in-law should end her reproductive career.'

A woman living in a simple household faces an entirely different set of problems compared to one living jointly with her parents-in-law. It is important to recall that a woman usually secedes from the joint household after a few years of marriage, by which time she attains motherhood and may have two or more children. By the time she establishes and manages her nuclear household efficiently, she bears one or two more children. It is at this time that she begins to contemplate termination of fertility. By this time she reaches the age of about 30. Many a time she thinks of getting herself sterilized. In Chapter 5 we have discussed a senior woman's responsibilities, multiple roles and greater interest in managing the household. Her primary interest lies in continuous hard work. Sterilization is not an easy decision when a woman is so preoccupied with the household. The overall responsibility of the household makes her think about all those issues which a mother-in-law raises before allowing her daughter-in-law to get sterilized. But once a senior woman decides to get herself sterilized, she somehow manages to seek her husband's support, which makes the decision less difficult for her than for a daughter-in-law living jointly in a complex household.

> Phooli, aged 35, initially discussed her desire to get sterilized with a friend who had prior experience. She then discussed the matter with her husband who agreed without much hesitation. Eventually, she got herself sterilized through laparoscopy in a family planning camp organized at Mogra. She chose an appropriate time—just a few months before she was to send her daugher away to her conjugal household for *muklāwo*.

Disapproval by the husband or the mother-in-law is not always an effective deterrent to a woman's final decision to get sterilized.

> Sugan, a young Charan woman in her late twenties and mother of three sons, always felt disgusted with her husband's indifference to her desire to get sterilized. He always diverted the issue and gave her false promises that her sterilization would be arranged. As time passed, she feared another conception. During one of her occasional stays at her parental home, she got herself sterilized, much to the displeasure of her husband and mother-in-law.
>
> Bhanwari, a middle-aged Harijan woman, mother of four sons and a daughter, felt exausted by the continuous bearing and rearing of children alongside regular wage work. Her husband, who lacked sympathy with her situation, always disapproved of her desire to get sterilized. One day she could not resist and went to the village camp for laparoscopy. On her return, she found her husband fuming in anger. He ordered her to leave his house and even hinted at divorcing her. It was only with the intervention of neighbours and friends that she could save herself from his wrath.

The women who acted in open defiance of their husbands' and in-laws' wishes were sure of their strength in the household. It derived partly from a few healthy surviving sons. This provided ample assurance to the mothers that their position in the household could not be easily destabilized.

> Sugan offered a vivid narrative of how she finally convinced her husband inspite of his strong reactions against her act: 'If we get a fourth son, how little land will each of the sons get! And

> if we had any daughter, how can we afford to marry her? The dowry expenses are rising day by day. Your salary is just sufficient to support the three boys and to educate them. Your opium addiction is no less expensive.' Sugan recalled that it took time before such an explanation finally pacified her husband's anger. She maintained that although the reaction of her husband and mother-in-law was hostile and painful (in the sense that she was not allowed to take proper rest after the operation), it did not last long. She summed up her gain, 'Whatever it may be, I am not reproducing like a goat.'

The foregoing description depicts the social resistance encountered by a woman in the process of deciding about sterilization. The tension between the woman's decision to get sterilized and the social resistance reveal significant principles of social organization within which fertility behaviour takes place. The process also highlights how the status of women ranges between moments of subordination and assertion in their attempts to control fertility. In other words, women have to submit to pressures from household elders on certain occasions, and are able to overthrow the pressures on other occasions.

It is significant to note that none of the sterilized women dared do so without making an effort to seek permission of the husband and household elders (cf. Caldwell *et al.* 1984 for this practice in South India). The few women who picked up courage to get themselves sterilized in open defiance of the husband and household elders may convey an impression that they were bold enough to take radical steps. But these women had overruled disapproval only after an overall asessment of their socially optimum fertility performance and their consequent status in the household. Only upon securing their expected fertility achievement did these women take to sterilization. It was accepted as an effective means of putting an end to their fertility career, which had reached an optimum point within the traditional norms. What appears to be a violation of fertility norms is in fact its reinforcement.

### *Responses to Sterilization*

The villagers' response to sterilization ranges from outright disapproval on the one hand to willing approval on the other. In between there are responses of ridicule, gossip, sacrasm, half-hearted acceptance, prudent indifference, etc. These responses are seldom arbitrary. They contain pointed references to people's experiences of fertility and child mortality. In most cases the responses come from the older people who have had greater exposure to high mortality during their younger days. Both over- and under-conformity to fertility norms evoke negative responses. Those who have got themselves sterilized after having just three or four children are believed to have ignored the child mortality of others in the village. To opt for sterilization in the face of imminent child mortality is to be blind.

Some reactions hardly assign a substantial reason against sterilization. Often the act of sterilization is criticized as unconventional. Such criticism, however, should not be taken merely at its face value. The disapproval is based on the elder's practical consciousness which is rarely expressed elaborately. A serious examination unfolds the imperatives of a subsistence- and labour intensive economy and high child mortality circumscribing the lives of people in Mogra. Getting sterilized after having three or four children is seen as refusal to recognize the real conditions. However, many young, and a few old, people are favourably disposed to sterilization, especially after a couple have had a few healthy grown up children.

> Bijoji, an old man owning a small patch of land, was perturbed when his only daughter gave birth to eight children in quick succession with two years' gap between each of them. He confided in me: 'It is no point having so many children without a stop. Three or four are enough. There are several means to put a stop these days. See how the whole house is littered.'

Those couples, all of whose children are surviving, give an impression of being more prolific than others. Having eight children with the eldest one about 16 years is exceeding the traditionally optimum fertility. With the eldest child reaching marriageable age, the household and other elders begin to get worried. They are anxious that such a couple cease to procreate any further.

> Kera, a 36-year-old Patel, had one son and a daughter. His first child came after a long wait of 12 years. Despite such an experience, he did not like the idea of having many children. He emphasized: 'I

will wait for two more years. May be, I'll get one more son. If I don't get a son in two years, I will put an end to this business (of procreation)'.

Devi, an elderly woman with five daughters, two sons and 15 grandchildren was convinced of the utility of sterilization, so much so that in her enthusiasm she willingly accompanied five women all the way to the hospital in Jodhpur city for operation. She looked after the five women and their infants for two days during their stay in the hospital. All these women were Devi's relatives. One of them was her daughter, while another her daughter-in-law.

Madi, a 62-year-old woman, was all in favour of getting her daughters-in-law sterilized. She arrived at this decision after her eldest daughter-in-law had three children and the next one, five.'

Kera, Devi and Madi have a few relatives in Jodhpur city. In addition, they have easy access to medical facilities as the doctor and nurse living in the village are their neighbours. Devi and Madi have several children and many more grandchildren. Neither of them has lost any grandchildren. The company of the doctor and the nurse has helped them favour sterilization. Such an approval of sterilization is not always forthcoming.

Several young persons make fun of those persons who get themselves sterilized.

Harji, a young man, ridiculed Bhera for his inability to control his wife from getting sterilized: 'Can't you even control your wife, or are you henpecked?' Choonoji, on the other hand, was rather indifferent and unconcerned about Bhera's wife's sterilization: 'It is their (Bhera's and his wife's) business. We can't stop it.' Vanji reacted in his peculiar way: 'This is in fashion these days.'

Even younger women drew caricatures of other women upon their strilization.

Veeri Darjee, a mother of four children, mimicked Ansi's awkward gait soon after her tubectomy in the city hospital. She also mimicked the gait through a play of her two fingers. She commented: 'It is so embarrassing to walk like that through the streets before so many elders. I would rather not get sterilized than walk awkwardly.'

As already discussed, sterilization is not a traditionally accepted practice, nor has it become very popular. Those getting sterilized have to face various ludicrous reactions. A pregnant woman's gait is seldom considered awkward, or ridiculed. Mimicking the changed gait after tubectomy is an expression of the cultural distinction of what is held as normal and abnormal.

A large number of people do not appreciate the new 'craze' for sterilization, and disapprove the technique disparagingly.

> Kesar, an old Charan woman with five sons and one daughter, did not approve of sterilization. She wanted her sons to have more than two sons each. Her desire got further strengthened as one of her sons could not produce a child despite more than a decade of marriage, and her only daughter lost her husband within two months of her mariage.' These experiences raised her doubts about sterilization and further strengthened her desire for high fertility.

Elderly parents become sensitive about fertility control, especially after the experience of prolonged childlessness of their married children. A large family is a matter of prestige for them.

> Bhoori, an old woman and mother of three sons and a daughter, had her own justifications against sterilization: 'I don't know what these younger women are up to. We never got ourselves mutilated like this. Mutilation for what? They are not better off than we. They can't sit back in a luxurious 'swing' (*hīndo*) with a foot resting on its edge and relax in a queenly way. Their life is no better than our's. What they derive out of such a step, only they know.' However, all her three daughters-in-law got sterilized after two of them had four survivng children each and the third had three with two surviving sons. Even her daughter underwent tubectomy after having three healthy sons. She fails to understand why her daughters-in-law and daughter should get sterilized.

As already mentioned, most elderly persons continue to fear high child mortality. Some of them took a tough position in not permitting younger women in their households to get sterilized.

> An old lady, addressed as Vaddi by most of her clan members, was so averse to sterilization that she would immediately become abusive whenever a reference was made to it. She would not only lose her temper and burst out emotionally while abusing people but also offer reasons for her negative reaction. During an interview she remarked: 'All those who are getting themselves sterilized are simply stupid. They do not understand any thing about life. They are going against God's will and life's wisdom. If the government claims to be powerful enough to stop more children

through those white-attired doctors, then why can't it provide children to those who are sterile and barren? It is only when it does so, can I believe in its superiority and power. Otherwise anyone can cut a 'cord' (*naḍ*) and commit the crime. Only the provider has the right to stop, those who can't provide have no such right. And what about bringing back to life those who die? What if your children die after your operation? Of what avail is the operation in such an eventuality? Of the three sons I had, two died in childhood and the last one died when he was old enough for *muklāwo*. He was my only hope. The doctors couldn't save him. I was left with no one in the world. Man is helpless before death. Then, where is the wisdom of getting sterilized? It is nothing but madness.'

Vaddi spoke in an intensely emotional way under the burden of her life experiences full of successive tragedies. She constantly carried the agony of losing all her family members and being left with none. To further substantiate her point she said: 'My husband's brother's daughter also had no children despite 20 years of marriage. The latter had a daughter who died within a few hours of birth and no child was born to her after that.' To her, children are hope; the more of them the greater the hope. Naturally, sterilization is termination of life and willing invitation for hopelessness. Vaddi's biography is replete with the wrath of child mortality which has left her with no strength even to tolerate others putting an end to their fertility.

Chidi, an old Harijan woman, strongly disapproved of the emerging trend towards fertility control. She was provoked when she overheard her daughter-in-law, a mother of four sons, being interviewed on the issue. She said: 'No one should get sterilized. There is no guarantee of life these days. Times are very adverse. There is a lot of sin spread all over the world. What can a woman do if all her children were to die after sterilization? In Tanavara (a neighbouring village) a Sargari (woman of Sargara caste) underwent tubectomy last year. She thought the three sons she had were enough for her. But as unfortunate as she is, two of her sons died of fever within two days of each other, and another died a month later. All the three healthy boys simply slipped out of her hands in less than a year of sterilizing. She couldn't help at all. She would only weep and wail. All this has driven her to mental illness and she talks incoherently. Her life is ruined. I will not permit my daughter-in-law to do such a thing. We will all share what we have. We will eat half instead of one (*Poori khāta ādi khaon*) and be satisfied rather than ruin ourselves by trying all kinds of nonsense. It is a sin to sterilize and the sinner is punished sooner or later. Sterilization leads to suffering.'

The adverse effects of sterilization are vividly recalled which deter several others from mustering courage to opt for it. Most of the elderly people disapprove of it partly from fear of post-surgical complications. The prevailing cosmology supports people's doubts about fertility-terminating measures, especially sterilization.

> Jhammu, a young woman in her twenties, was apprehensive about her future incarnation because of sterilization. 'So many people have told me that sterilization amounts to torturing all those beings who were destined to be born to a woman. Denying them entry in this world does not absolve the woman. She will have to bear all the remaining children in her next incarnation. There is no respite from this. One has to finish one's task before attaining *gati*.'

The apprehensions and premonitions pertain not only to some of the actual fertility experiences of people and of those who got themselves sterilized, but also to the religious and moral notions of procreation and of karma that a couple is destined to fulfill. Some of the elderly take the cosmology more seriously than others in not permitting their young daughters and daughters-in-law to get sterilized. As sterilization is a relatively recent, unconventional technique, the elderly rarely welcome it. Factors such as fear of child mortality, post-operative debility, and interference in religious and moral precepts, constitute the mixed reactions to sterilization.

## *Conclusion*

As none of the modern contraceptive and sterilization techniques has indigenous cultural moorings, the village people experience a variety of tensions, uncertainties and indecision in adopting them. The family planning techniques are definite indices of change but have not radically altered the continuities in the norms of fertility behaviour.

People's acceptance of FPP is partial, and is mediated by prevailing norms and values, resulting in selection of its various components. The selective acceptance is only a fraction of the total package, and is conditioned by people's real experiences in the handling of family planning techniques and consequent accumulated memory. A technique is accepted insofar as it facilitates the norms of fertility regulation. The acceptance of sterilization in no way contravenes traditional norms regarding the onset and termination of fertility, the socially expected number of children, and the status of the woman as bearer of children. The compulsion of strenuous physical work has a crucial role in deciding the choice of the method of sterilisation. Since laparoscopy does not require prolonged absence from work in and outside the household, and is accessible in the vicinity of the village, and sometimes even within it, it is preferred to tubectomy. People's indifference to some of the components of the package is not an indication of their ignorance or non-response as is observed by numerous KAP surveys. On the contrary, people's indifference to many FPP measures is a result of their rejection of them. What KAP surveys call indifference is the other name for irrelevance to people.

Even in the case of villagers having vital links with the city, acceptance of sterilization has not contravened prescribed norms of fertility. In earlier chapters, we discussed the fertility behaviour of those holding urban jobs and/or living in urban areas or of those commuting to the city regularly. They have accepted fertility control only after achieving the socially optimum number of children. Even if a technique reinforces prevailing fertility practices, it is not always accepted unquestioningly by one and all. The responses of the people vary from outright opprobrium to quiet acceptance. This is the way FPP is locally unpackaged. Only those convenient components gain gradual acceptance among some people. Also, only the constituents which conform to the pressures and prescriptions of traditional society find a place in the village society, and of course invite mixed responses.

CHAPTER 8

# Conclusion

This study has tried to provide an interpretive account of fertility behaviour in the village society of Mogra. It has analysed fertility behaviour in the context of social structure, people's behaviour, meanings and perceptions, and institutional mechanisms, i.e., customs, rituals and ceremonies. It has identified how various institutional mechanisms operate to enable couples to continue child bearing and rearing for long periods during their fertility career. A holistic perspective has led to an integrated view of the village community and its functioning with particular reference to fertility behaviour as it is carried on routinely. This account is based mainly on the method of intensive fieldwork, which one believes is fruitful for a more adequate grasp of the complexity of fertility behaviour. The fieldwork method, involving unstructured interviews, participant observation, case studies, village census, retrospective fertility histories of all ever married women, and other relevant documentation, has made possible a dense description of fertility behaviour in Mogra.

Departing from the divide between subjective and objective frameworks in fertility studies, the present study links objective conditions of life with people's subjective orientations, including values and norms of fertility behaviour. In this light, special attention is given to the modalities of regulation and control of fertility behaviour throughout the fertility career of husband-wife couples. Giddens' (1984) concept of the 'duality of structure' is a useful tool in overcoming the conceptual divide between objective conditions of life influencing fertility outcomes on the one hand, and subjective orientations affecting fertility behaviour on the other.

Duality means that objective conditions and people's subjective orientations together constitute the medium as well as the outcome of recursive social practices.

Contrary to the position of socio-economic and macro-structural studies which view couples as mere subjects in the service of social structure, couples in Mogra are in active and regular interaction with the social structure. In other words, the couple and the social sturcture are an interacting whole. To put it differently, fertility behaviour has to be analysed in the context of the dialectics between social values and objective reality. A complex set of factors come into play in this dialectics. An analysis of the cosmology of fertility and of family ideology reveals the underlying conceptions and values regarding sterility, fecundity, childbirth, sons and daughters, etc. These are crucial in organizing couples' fertility behaviour within the framework of the objective conditions of life.

A comprehensive view of fertility behaviour reveals that it is an integral part of the complex totality of social behaviour. Though the present study is focussed on fertility, it has discussed other aspects of population as well. Mortality and migration, the other two of the three important population processes, receive attention insofar as they impinge upon and contribute to the understanding of fertility behaviour. The incidences of infant and child mortality, and people's perceptions and responses to them are discussed at length. The relationship of immigrants and emigrants with the village, their status, role and impact on the social life of the people, especially on their fertility behaviour, are discussed.

In the discussion on childbirth, child mortality, and fertility regulation and control, fertility behaviour has been placed in the context of the developmental process of the household and the related fertility career of the couple. This process and career is kept in view throughout to see how couples, especially women, manage and organize their fertility performance while keeping in mind various currents and processes during different phases of their fertility career. The concept of fertility career of a couple is critical to the understanding of the social regulation of fertility. The concept of the developmental process of the household (Shah 1973) clearly has heuristic value in the understanding of the phases of development of the fertility career of a couple. While the fertility career of a couple and the household go through phases of progression and regression, one cannot always bring correspondence between the phases that they go through. The progressive phase of a fertility career begins with the marriage of a couple. The various processes in the social organization of childbirth indicate and facilitate the progression of the fertility career. Mortality of a child and a spouse indicate regression. The couple's fertility career culminates with the cessation of procreation. This is closely linked with the marriage of their children and the onset of the latter's fertility career.

The career graph of fertility indicates the developmental phases of progression (in terms of childbirth and child survival, culminating in older couples ceasing to produce children and the younger ones beginning their fertility careers) and regression (through child mortality). The concept of fertility career helps to view fertility behaviour as a process rather than a static reality. This does not, however, imply that fertility career is cyclical in development. Although it has a specific beginning (with marriage), marked socially in the life of a couple, the extent of progression and the precise sequence of its phases are not predetermined, nor is it identical to all couples. A couple's fertility career may go forward or backward during its course. A woman's marriage marks the beginning of her fertility career. Its progression takes place with the conception of her first child. Her age at first childbirth tends to influence the future course of her fertility career. Child mortality is a regression in her fertility career. Her marital status is crucial to her fertility. The number and sex of children born, child mortality, and consequent child survival have a great bearing on her total fertility performance. The marriage of her children and the onset of the latter's fertility careers leads to the termination of her own.

Culture and social values play an important role in the fertility career of a woman. Incorporation of a woman in her conjugal household and birth of child(ren) are culturally determined. The customs of marriage, in particular, those of remarriage of widowed and divorced women, have implications for women's fertility. Among the upper castes where remarriage is not permitted, women endure the stigma of barrenness throughout their lives. On the other hand, castes permitting remarriage have positive implications for fertility.

The analysis of fertility behaviour in Mogra questions some of the prevailing views in demographic research. Human fertility is culture-specific. To put it in the words of some demographers, fertility behaviour is not 'natural' but 'target'-oriented, i.e., it does not follow an impulsive and unhindered course (see Handwerker 1986). The data from Mogra also reveals that fertility behaviour is socially regulated and not primarily instinctive as is believed to be the case in pre-transitional societies i.e., traditional societies where fertility decline has not begun. It emerges from indigenous modes of fertility regulation and control in Mogra that rural people are not lacking in reason and rationality. Far from being instinctive, fertility behaviour is governed by forethought and folk wisdom.

The KAP studies, which constitute a substantial segment of demographic studies on fertility in India, have based their observations and correlations through the use of survey methods. They have put forward the view that rural people are neither aware of modern methods of contraception nor inclined to use them. The data from Mogra and other parts of India belies this view. The people of Mogra resort to a judicious mix of modern and indigenous methods of fertility control. Modern techniques are accepted insofar as they dovetail with indigenous practices.

Several studies have tried to establish a relationship between fertility behaviour and a given family type. However, these studies have given little consideration to the developmental process of the household. Few studies have shown the relevance to fertility behaviour of the age of couples and their position and stage in the developmental process of the household. The tendency has been to locate fertility behaviour in a straight-jacket dichotomy of nuclear and joint family—a dichotomy found to be inadequate, if not meaningless, in the study of family in India.

This study has shown that the critical norm in the formation of the household in Mogra is the residential unity of patrikin and their wives, which entails the norm of patrivirilocality. A large number of couples in Mogra practise this norm. Those who get separated from joint households to form their own simple ones do so after having lived patrivirilocally for a considerable period of time. Most of these couples have a few children before they are separated from the joint household. Therefore, critical to our understanding is the way in which a woman transits through different types of household compositions during her fertility career. Significantly, her children are born and brought up partly in the joint and partly in the nuclear household. The context of the developmental process of the household is thus crucial in understanding fertility behaviour.

Some studies of fertility argue that lack of communication between spouses in tratidional joint families enhances fertility. But we have seen how in Mogra couples in nuclear households who are supposed to enjoy a greater degree of inter-personal communication as well as couples in joint households who are supposed to lack it have almost the same number of children.

A widely prevalent view in fertility studies posits a relation between women's age at marriage and fertility, namely, that those who marry early have a longer marital duration and scope for higher fertility. The data from Mogra does not support this view. Irrespective of their age at marriage and some variations in marital duration, most mothers in the culmination stage of their fertility careers have nearly the same number of children. Also, women married before the age of 15 and those married between 16 and 20 years of age have little variation in number of children born. The period between marriage and first childbirth is slightly longer for those women married by the age of 15 than for those married later, which evens out the effect of age at marriage on fertility. Exceptional cases in this regard are usually the ones affected adversely by the process of regression (due to widowhood, divorce, child mortality and sterility) in their fertility careers.

In several demographic studies, gainful employment (income-generating activity of women outside the house) is viewed as enhancing the status of women and lowering their fertility. However, the reality is different and more complex. First of all, marriage, motherhood and birth of children, especially of sons, confer social status on women. In other words, status improves with fertility and not with gainful employment. This gives security to women in and outside the household. The progression of a woman's fertility career steps up her status further. Childbirth and child survival confer honour on the mother. Motherhood integrates the daughter-in-law into the conjugal household. A mother with four or five surviving children (including sons) is held in high esteem as compared to a childless woman. Marriage of children and birth of grandchildren further enhance the parents' esteem. The negative sanction on barrenness supports the high social value of motherhood. Barrenness is a curse. A barren woman is often ridiculed, at times abused, and is under the constant fear of a possible second marriage by her husband. The pathos of barrenness in comparison to well-being and prosperity of fecundity in Mogra society is quite striking.

Secondly, it needs to be discussed whether women's work on family farms and home-based assistance in income-generating activities in rural society are gainful employment or not. Moreover, the question that needs to be raised in this context is: has gainful employment any bearing on fertility behaviour? In Mogra there are castes among whom women are confined to the household, while among other castes women work outside the household, either on their own family farms or of others. Between the two, the social milieu of Mogra does not impute high social value to gainfully-employed women. In fact, the *purdah*-observing upper caste women who are not gainfully employed are looked upon as enjoying higher status. The social values of rural society in India are not in correspondence with those of urban, industrial societies of the west. The tendency to transpose the values and concepts of western industrial society onto rural Indian society in fertility studies by demographers has resulted in ill-founded correlations such as that between gainful employment and status of women.

A major debate relates to the value and cost of children. Once again, the existing views put forward by some demographers and economists suffer from an urban bias. A good number of studies by micro-economists attribute value to children in the context of costs and benefits. The well-known argument, 'a baby or a car', put foward by Becker (1960) equates children to consumer durables. The micro-economists do not, however, take into consideration the unacknowledged factors behind fertility. In other words, they ignore the fact that before having a child a couple seldom calculate only in economic terms every aspect of their behaviour that contributes to fertility. The attitudes toward children and child rearing practices reveal the cultural irrelvance of such economic reductionism in Mogra.

In contrast to Becker's views, Caldwell's (1982: 333–61) theory of wealth flows is a breakthrough in the understanding of fertility. He explains that reduction of fertility in urban and industrial societies occurs with changes in family values and morality. Couples in such societies tend to spend most of their economic and other resources within their nuclear family. The path to enhancement of status in such a society is by spending one's resources not on the wider network of relatives but on members of the nuclear family. The wealth flows (all the money, goods, services and guarantees that one person provides to another) in these societies, he maintains, is channelled from parents to children, and not from children to parents. Parents thus prefer to have fewer rather than larger number of children. The fewer the children, the lesser the expenses on them. Caldwell's theory moves away from the naive thesis of economic calculations of couples, i.e., making a choice between having a consumer durable or a baby.

Significantly, Caldwell breaks away from the conventional preoccupation of treating industrial and non-industrial societies as undifferentiated. He makes a distinction between traditional societies where services play a predominant role as opposed to modern societies which are commodity centred. Yet Caldwell's brilliant analysis does not unravel the invisibility of the substantial contributions made by rural parents to their children. His formulation of wealth flows does not overcome urban bias entirely. He too tends to analyse wealth flows in traditional societies from the vantage point of modern industrial society. The argument is that in urban societies parents spend liberally on their children, while those in pre-transitional societies rarely incur similar expenditure. He overlooks the fact that parents in traditional societies expend on children in invisible ways.

In Mogra, as elsewhere in the region, parents make conscious efforts not only to protect but also to increase the land, house site, cattle and other property to be used and inherited by their children for earning their livelihood (cf. Lorimer 1954). While the nature of property held by parents to be passed on to their children may vary in relation to family type and caste, the fact remains that children are the subject of parents' motivation for an active social life. Childless parents feel a vacuum in their life. For example, upper caste parents work towards bequeathing to their children land, house, jewellery and such other property. In contrast, parents from lower caste and an economically poor background impart to their children skills such as blacksmithy and pottery, and access to common property resources, in addition to whatever material resources they have. Parents also transfer the symbolic honour and prestige gradually accumulated by them through conformity and fulfilment of numerous social, familial and kinship obligations at various stages of their life cycle—efforts and contributions which often go unnoticed.

In the rural society of Mogra an individual's identity is submerged into that of the household and family. An individual's status is closely tied to that of the household. The members of the household, whether children or adults, are expected to maintain the status of the household and enhance its prosperity. Children not only have an economic value but are also important politically. They contribute to the enlargement of lineage, kinship, caste and neighbourhood ties. Even a daughter contributes to her natal household's status through affinal linkages. It is in this context that motherhood gains critical importance in women's lives. The world view of the family in Mogra, which underplays individualism in favour of the collectivity of the household, is sustained by religious beliefs and practices.

Agriculture in Mogra is labour intensive, drawing mainly upon household labour. Members of the household support, and are generally involved in, each other's activities. They are engaged in diverse occupations. Frequently one member of the household does another's tasks in his/her absence, or helps in doing them. All these economic activities place emphasis on labour inputs. The multiplicity of tasks and the labour involved in them places a high premium on children. Parents receive contributions from children not only in terms of immediate labour available but also see clearly their potential contribution to keeping the household going in the ups and downs of life. To have a large household and a wide network of relatives is to have a support structure to fall back upon in adversity.

The incidence of high child mortality and the fear of losing children motivates couples to have more than the optimum number of children they would like to have. Fertility is controlled only after having the socially expected number of children. If a woman continues to bear children even after crossing the age of 40 because of her having lost several children, she is not scorned at. On the other hand, her efforts and condition receive sympathy. Again, the cases of women who have suffered the death of several children are frequent reminders to younger couples to negotiate the objective reality of child mortality by nurturing views favouring high fertility. The fear syndrome of child mortality promotes a culture of high fertility. The death of a child is mourned collectively, and the accumulated pool of knowledge influences couples to reckon with mortality in their own fertility performance.

The premium placed on the unity of patrikin, the collectivity of the household, and the social value of children nurture a culture where motherhood is made attractive and covetous. However, motherhood is not appreciated throughout a woman's life. Honour and shame get attached to motherhood according to age and stage in the fertility career. Social norms of fertility behaviour are at once constraining and enabling. The society around the mother actively monitors her fertility performance throughout her fertility career.

Childbirth does not have an easy passage in the life of a mother. But childbirth is buttressed and attendant pains are lessened and smoothened in various ways by relatives and members of the household. The immediate relatives' close attention to the comforts of the mother accentuates the significance of the event of childbirth. For example, the household ignores all gender-specific rules governing labour, leisure, rest and valued food in favour of a *japaiti*. The mother is made to realize in more ways than one that childbirth is not just a personal event but also a social one. The various gifts and rituals, including the observance of pollution by a prescribed set of relatives, reinforce the social value of childbirth. Rituals, appreciation and gifts act as positive sanctions, motivating women to abide by social norms. The disgrace attached to sterility and barrenness instils fear among women, and motivates them to enter motherhood. A rich repository of proverbs, maxims, anecdotes, folk tales and folk music conditions perceptions and rationalizes the social prescriptions of fertility behaviour.

As said earlier, there is no unconditional approval of motherhood. It is a matter of shame for an elderly couple to have children after the marriage of their grown-up children. Mothers having children at a later stage in life face negative sanctions through disapproval and ridicule. A pregnant grandmother is subjected to a lot of harsh criticism and is looked down upon as bringing dishonour.

The trend of high fertility in Mogra does not mean that there is little effort on the part of couples to arrest the process of reproduction. While one set of conditions promotes fertility, another set curtails the mother's reproductive role. It is not uncommon to find mothers arresting procreation, especially during the latter phase of their fertility career. The eventuality of death of the aged in the household and the attendant expenditure on mortuary rituals, religious rituals, children's marriages and such other occasions are considerations for a mother to slow down or even stop further procreation. But these considerations figure at a later stage in the procreative career of a mother. The stage at which she begins to take cognizance of these considerations is also related to the developmental process of the household, as for example, her becoming mother-in-law and grandmother. These considerations begin to have a bearing on her ability to stop procreation. Above all, women gain a good measure of freedom and control over their own lives at this stage. But the more important aspect is the way in which objective conditions are perceived and interpreted for fertility behaviour. For instance, economic considerations are interpreted by the mother of a few teenaged children in such a way that it encourages her to restrict fertility. But the same mother, though somewhat aware of these considerations at an earlier stage of her fertility career, proves her motherhood and thus enhances her status.

Interventions by social institutions do constrain but seldom without some room for couples to exercise their ingenuity and volition. For instance, a couple having four children and another having six are both behaving within the permissible range of normative fertility. The fact that the optimum number of children fall in the range of three to six itself provides inbuilt flexibility.

In other words, if a couple has four and not five or six children, it is not considered to be deviant. What is important is that people in Mogra do not want a very large number, say eight or more, of surviving children. The cases of termination of fertility through sterilization by some women soon after having the socially minimum number of children reflect the adaptability of social norms. The acceptance of modern means of fertility control in open defiance of elders reveals resort to deviant strategies, though within the traditional set up. Individual idiosyncracies in strategy come up and are met with different responses in and outside the household. In such situations, discrepancies are minimized through manoeuvres and compromises which help to reproduce the social structure in which fertility takes place, and maintain its continuity. Although such deviations are still a negligible minority, they seem to forecast a future trend.

It is relevant in this context to reflect on the entry of modern institutions, such as the school, dispensary and urban employment of a few villagers, and their impact on rural life. Some changes are emerging, particularly new ideas about marriage and man-woman relations, which are coming from the media, social reforms, urban exposure, impact of immigrants, and so on, and are having an influence on fertility behaviour, especially in reducing birth intervals and acceptance of sterilization. But not all new ideas are accepted unquestioningly. While urban employment is held in high esteem, the school has gained only partial acceptance. The methods of contraception promoted by FPP are received with a great measure of caution. Time-hallowed indigenous methods are tried before modern methods of family planning are given a try. Significantly modern methods of contraception are practised only after couples have had the socially prescribed number of children. Not all methods of modern family planning have received uncritical acceptance. For example, data shows that only laparoscopy has received some acceptance compared to other methods of fertility termination, primarily because of its suitability to the arduous labour that Mogra women engage in.

The selective acceptance of FPP and modern measures of fertility control becomes meaningful only because it has been understood in the context of traditional institutional practices and techniques of fertility control prevalent in Mogra. Our data suggests that modern fertility control measures are mediated by local structures of institutions, values and attitudes. In view of the above understanding, it is important for any policy to acquire knowledge about indigenous and traditional social institutions. For fruitful policy formulation and intervention, it is critical to have an integrated view of a given society.

An in-depth understanding of the objective conditions of life and people's subjective orientation in Mogra has been possibile through intensive and rigorous fieldwork. It has enabled access to social, cultural and symbolic aspects of fertility behaviour, including norms, values, customs, conventions, proverbs, maxims, anecdotes, rituals, appreciation, criticism and cosmology. It has reiterated the importance of the fieldwork method in achieving the above account of fertility behaviour, revealing complexity scarcely revealed by survey research of this intimate aspect of human behaviour.

In identifying processes, including institutional ways and means, influencing fertility behaviour, the present research could not pay adequate attention to processes involved in gradually bringing the change in fertility behaviour. There exist regularized relations of autonomy and dependence between couples and collectivities in the interactional nexus. The innovation in fertility behaviour emerging through various modes in the interface between autonomy and dependence could be explored more systematically. The cases of women who were inclined towards sterilization and who managed to go through it indicate an area for further study.

It would be worthwhile to explore the concept of fertility career of a couple for further understanding of social regulation of fertility behaviour and the institutional mechanisms through which it operates in society.

The emphasis of this study has been on women. The data pertaining to subjective orientations and ways in which strategies for organizing and regulating fertility are evolved are obtained largely from women. Although men have not been totally ignored, they have not been covered sufficiently. It would be of value to explore their role and perspective on fertility behaviour.

# APPENDICES

APPENDIX I

# A Note on Fieldwork

In Chapter 1, I have discussed the broad methodological approach adopted for the present study. Here I describe the nature of my fieldwork in Mogra.

Studying one's own society has advantages as well as disadvantages. Fieldwork in Mogra was no exception. I encountered challenges similar to those faced by Unni (1979) and Joshi (1979) in studying their societies. Unlike my first study which was confined to the Patel caste, and the second which was not a prolonged one, though covering all the castes, the present study posed problems I had not encountered earlier. As I carried the mark of membership of the Patel caste, I had to secure for myself an acceptable image before the other castes.

While there were certain advantages in selecting Mogra, I also faced a number of problems. Here's how I tried to overcome them.

I managed to get residential accommodation in Mogra as soon as I began the study. I got my father's ancestral house (uninhabitated most of the time) cleaned, and made arrangements to stay there. However, staying in a particular caste area created problems of access to other caste areas (cf. Beteille and Madan 1975; and Srinivas *et al.* 1979). Being a Patel and living in a Patel street had initially meant more access to a certain part of the village than to others. Nevertheless, both Patels as well as non-Patels initially felt puzzled due to my frequent visits to them.

Entry into untouchable households turned out to be a difficult task. It put my skills as a fieldworker to real test. Members of both higher and lower castes expressed strong disapproval when I was seen approaching an untouchable household. Once a woman from Kareegar (carpenter) caste spotted me at the entrance of a Bhangi's (scavenger's) house. She dragged me away forcibly because only members of Bhangi caste (lowest in caste hierarchy) are supposed to enter a Bhangi house. Much later, I once dared sneak into the Bhangi house after dusk for a brief period. Generally I had to sit outside an untouchable's house, on the *chauntari* (elevated platform on either or both sides of the house), while talking to the inmates. At odd hours, like late evening or scorching afternoon, I used to slip into their homes. To my pleasant surprise, they felt happy and honoured by the entry of a person like me from a higher caste into their homes. However, due to rigid observance of commensal taboos, they never offered me food or drink. This in turn pre-empted a probable strong reaction from the upper castes. Such a fear was not entirely imaginary, for I had read about Chakravarty's (1979) similar experience in a village in north-eastern Rajasthan.

My entry into homes of higher castes, especially those of Charans and Rajputs, was not easy either. Many of their men knew me through my father. But I was relatively new to their women, particularly the younger ones. The older women had heard of my father who, unlike other Patels, had sent his daughters to school and college, and was laughed at till the village people learnt of my teaching profession. The Charan women would stare at me and look questioningly when I entered their homes.

I maintained a polite and unassuming posture unexpected of urban salaried job holders. To the villagers I was a 'highly educated person' employed in Delhi, which they considered the most important city in India. My friendly approach appealed to them and helped me in gaining access to all people. To their surprise, I behaved quite unlike the educated government officials they had known. I would always initiate conversation, because this was considered an act of humility on the part of an official coming from outside. I upheld their self-respect and made them feel important. I interviewed them in a manner which made them feel comfortable. I always avoided sitting on a chair, cot, gunny bag or mattress which they readily brought for me. Instead I preferred to sit or stand wherever the respondents were, though they rarely allowed me to do this. My equalitarian behaviour, which they did not expect from a person with my education and job, had a winning influence.

I had practised the use of local modes of greeting like *Ram Ram Sa* (literally, 'In the glory of Rama'), 'How are you?', and 'How do you do?' as a pretext to create space for interviews. As is customary for married daughters, I used to bow my head before elderly persons to receive their blessings. This gesture before elders and my distributing sweets to children were much appreciated. In the eyes of the higher caste people I could gain acceptability due to my speaking in the local dialect, which to them was refined and more cultured by village standards. My speech carried the imprint of my urban upbringing which was similar to that of the higher castes.

Having overcome the initial hesitations, I had little problem of access to upper caste homes in the village. The Charan women enjoyed the interviews so much that they did not want them to end. An interview was a pleasant diversion for them, particularly in the background of their custom of *purdo* which restricted them to their homes most of the time. Later, it became difficult for me to take their leave. While working with the Charan women, on several occasions, I was affectionately forced to retire in their homes at night rather than go to spend the night in the house where I lived all by myself. Their insistence on my staying with them was a blessing in disguise. I could observe them more closely at odd hours. I availed similar opportunities in several other homes too. We had early dinner (common in Mogra) and usually several Charan women assembled in one of the houses to gossip, especially to spend some time with me, after dinner. It was easier for them to move about under the cover of darkness. At other times, particularly during summer, women got together in the street and sang hymns until mignight. In between the hymns there was always some gossip about the world. Occasionally, a few non-Charan women also joined the group, which further enriched my understanding of inter-caste relations in the village. In order to secure greater access to various caste groups, I had managed to have informants from different castes.

Initially, the villagers' were afraid and distrustful on seeing me with a questionnaire ('paper and pen' to most of them). From my earlier fieldwork experience I had learnt that questioning them with 'paper and pen' made them think that I was deputed by the government (Rāj), by Mrs Indira Gandhi (the then Prime Minister) to gather some important information about them, either for extra taxation or such other purpose. They thought I was sent from Delhi to get reliable information through my links with Mogra.

Learning from previous experience, I decided not to begin the census survey for a few weeks. In the meantime, I not only ventured out to socialize with people, but also invited several school and college going boys for informal conversation. This was appreciated by the people. Several parents even requested me to provide some guidance to their children regarding education. Through informal sessions with them, I explained the nature of my fieldwork in simple terms. I discussed with them the kind of data I needed and how my work would proceed. I explained my research by comparing it with the decennial census. As most of them did not know that a census took place every 10 years, they easily believed my study to be another census survey. This was further reinforced in people's minds by the school boys who explained to them my work in one word—census. These boys were gradually convinced that the kind of work I had undertaken in the village was for the purpose of writing a Ph.D. dissertation, and was in no way inimical to the interests of the village and its people. The boys' initial inhibition was gradually overcome with my daily contact and interaction with them.

The school boys were instrumental in creating an impression in the minds of people, especially of their parents and close relatives, that my fieldwork was benign and would cover every household in the village without discrimination. The household census, I now realize, was a blessing. After having convinced the students, I finalized the census schedule and prepared myself to administer it.

My census work benefitted from the willing assistance provided by a few school boys as well as a few elderly persons. They helped me in locating respondents and introduced me to them. They were effective in encouraging people to open up and also to help them recall and cross check certain information or details pertaining to childbirth, death, age at wedding, marriage, separation of the household, partition of property, income, land, etc. Within a few days, almost the entire village was favourably disposed towards my household census. The people were no longer apprehensive of the questions I raised and of the sight of paper and pen in my hand. However, people's fear was only an initial problem I overcame. Many others were to follow.

Some mischievous children caused a minor inconvenience during the initial few months of fieldwork. All children were curious about me and my activities. A few of them always accompained me wherever I went. They entered my respondents' homes along with me without any hesitation and had to be driven away with difficulty. The respondents yelled at these children without inviting adverse reactions from their parents.

I faced certain limitations in the field as a woman. My role as a fieldworker demanded violation of certain rules to be observed by women in Mogra. As a woman, I was not expected to talk to men freely and put questions to them (cf. Bellwinkel 1979 and Gupta 1979 for their fieldwork experiences on this issue). I had to reckon with the fact that I was a woman in a male-dominated society. My interviews often stretched across several hours, which seemed to people 'useless gossip' or 'extra socializing'. This was contrary to the dominant image of a woman. Gradually people began to feel that I was genuinely interested in befriending them, and they reconciled to my 'gossiping'.

My visiting people's homes throughout the day instead of remaining within the home was perceived as 'aimless wandering' and contrary to women's behaviour in Mogra. Women do move out in the village but seldom without a purpose. And the purpose is usually confined to routine tasks like fetching water and fuel, tending cattle, etc., when women often meet others. Gossip sessions with close neighbours or women in the street, however, is an accepted part of the routine that takes place only once or twice a day. Women generally refrain from visiting people farther than the immediate neighbourhood.

In contrast, I moved out quite uninhibitedly in the entire village. Only gradually did I secure tacit approval for my 'odd' behaviour. In general, the village people evolved a rationale for my behaviour, by thinking that I was deputed for the purpose of inspecting the village. In addition, my appearance and routine conduct convinced them to give me such a concession. I was consciously conforming to most of the customary norms, particularly those that did not interfere with my research. Although I wore a saree which was strikingly different in size and style than that of the village women, I always covered my head with it in the same way as other women do, as a mark of respect to senior men and women. I refrained from using sun glasses or an umbrella despite the scorching heat and strong dusty desert winds. This made my appearance more acceptable to people and even stray dogs (that usually turn aggressive towards unfamiliar people). These encounters in the field enabled me incidentally to learn a great deal about normative behaviour guided by principles of caste, seniority and gender.

It was not much of a problem to remain in the company of women most of the time, but prolonged discussions with men by a woman were considered undesirable. As a result, I had to spend most of the time with women. Of course, a few male informants were crucial for the study. Sex segregation is more strict among Charan and Rajput castes whose women observe *purdo*. Among other castes, men were present off and on during the time I sat with women in their homes or in the street. In fact, men preferred to talk to me while I sat among women, mostly to make their presence felt. Some even requested that I teach something to the women to make them literate. A few male informants, other than school-going and the college drop-out boys, played a significant role in fieldwork. Certain concessions in heterosexual interaction were made to me due to the importance which people attributed to my status as a married daughter of Mogra, and as being highly educated and employed despite belonging primarily to a society where girls are rarely sent to school. But all this helped very little in eliciting responses from men over issues pertaining to fertility and contraception, except that I was able to discuss with a few men the issues of sterilization, child health and education.

My prior familiarity with the field had certain disadvantages too. I had to think twice before putting several questions to the people, because they expected me to know about them. They ridiculed me for my ignorance when I enquired about certain details of wedding rituals, cooking recipes, child care, etc. I felt embarrassed to express my inability to recognize people I was supposed to know well. They were either very prominent in the village social life or belonged to my father's lineage. I would upset parents if I did not recognize their children. My inability to recognize people whom I had met during the earlier fieldwork, or who were not very distant relatives, conveyed to them my lack of a sense of proximity towards them. Of course, I was excused for my clumsiness by comments like, 'She has never lived here', 'She is getting acquainted', etc.

My house in the field was expected to be open to all throughout the day. As other houses are usually open during day time, mine was to be even more so, as people were genuinely inquisitive about me and my lifestyle. Adults as well as children from the neighbourhood were usually present whenever I was at home. I was hardly left alone for most part of the day. After a couple of weeks, the number of people gradually thinned down, but never was I given an opportunity to be all by myself even for a few hours. I requested people to leave the house while I bathed. Children and women invariably had difficulty in understanding why they should. They expected me to bathe without turning them out. Besides, people liked to watch while I cooked my meals. A lone person cooking meals for herself/himself is a sign of misfortune and destitution in Mogra. Although people knew I was not destitute, it was an unusual sight for them to see me cooking for myself. They also preferred me to share my meal with them. Initially I was unprepared to offer meals to the several persons sitting in my house as I cooked only for myself. Later I began to cook larger quantities and offered them as well. Of course, they too invitied me to meals occasionally. Throughout the fieldwork period spread over more than a year, I was not allowed to bolt the door even during siesta in the unbearably hot summer afternoons. People, especially children, were always waiting to enter my house the moment I unlocked it on my return from someone's home. A procession of children was usually with me during my visits to various houses.

Inquiry was not my sole prerogative. While I was trying to know about the village and its people, they were trying to know about me. It was a two-way process of learning. The village people wanted to know about me, my family life, my kinsmen, job, income, etc. They were in general quite inquisitive and observant about me. I was warned by several people not to visit a particular Patel household whose senior-most woman was believed to be a witch. The frankness with which they enquired about my personal life was enough to give culture shock to an American sociologist who once acompanied me to the village. His first comment in astonishment was, 'In America you cannot ask personal questions, especially pertaining to income, even in your third or fourth meeting with a person, let alone of a stranger. I was feeling quite uneasy while both of you (I and the truck driver who gave us a lift) were talking about your salary.'

In addition to their curiosity about me, people had evolved a certain way of defining me (cf. Minocha 1979 for an elaboration of this point). They thought I was a highly placed government official in Delhi. Many parents wanted me to arrange jobs for their school and college drop-out sons. Many others wanted to borrow money from me, sometimes large amounts running into tens of thousands of rupees. They would frequently inquire about my salary, and however small an amount I stated it to be, it appeared a huge amount to them. They calculated my expenses in accordance with theirs, and assessed the remaining as my saving, which they thought they could borrow. One of them calculated my annual saving in his own way, and announced that it could purchase a tractor every year. He wanted me to lend him a year's savings to enable him to buy a tractor. The villagers also requested me to take patients to city hospitals for treatment, and to intervene in various government offices in the city where their applications or other papers lay stuck. They thought that my representing them would either expedite the work free of cost, or at least lessen the amount of bribe to be paid. I was expected to give medicines, sweets, small gifts and cash (mostly to children). A few people desired a gift for every one of them for information on them. They had somehow sensed that the fieldwork and the report on it would help me in my career, and since they were actively contributing towards it, they thought it right that I share the benefit with them.

I did respond to some of these expectations. I took patients to the city hospital for treatment. One of them came to the hospital specifically to know about family planning methods. I gave sweets and small cash gifts, mostly to children. But I never got myself involved in lending money, being apprehensive of the consequences of money-lending. I knew the value of the proverb, 'Lend money and lose a friend.' I realized that asceptic research was not possible for a participant observer. One had to decide in favour of pragmatic instead of puristic fieldwork, in the words of Srinivas *et al.* (1979: 7–10).

A few expectations of the villagers had to be fulfilled without losing the goal of research. I was often prodded to take sides in favour of or against a person or a household. Such situations were not unusual across caste, age, sex and kin ties. Along with warmth and tolerance there existed jealousy, criticism, humour and sarcasm in Mogra. Fortunately, I managed to keep myself away from excessive involvement in people's quarrels which would have made data collection nearly impossible. Of course, it was much easier for me to encourage them to talk freely when they confided in me.

The extremely hostile weather conditions in summer and other tribulations of a backward village in a third world country need not be mentioned here in detail. The abundance of simplicity and warmth in everyday behaviour, and the safety and affection provided by the people neutralized many physical inconveniences.

While conducting in-depth interviews, I not only visited people's houses but also walked along with groups of men, and more often, of girls and adult women going to fetch water or fuel or on other errands. I met people at the bus stop, temples, shrines, construction sites, shops, the dispensary, pond, well, handpumps, *chauntaries* of houses, etc. In addition, I met people in the homes of oil pressers, tailors, barbers, carpenters, adult and non-formal education instructors, and of those who had guests visiting them. Several people congregated in these places and at certain junctions and crossings of streets and engaged themselves in prolonged gossip. Some people were almost regular visitors to these sites. I identified several key men informants in these places, while I had identified most key women informants during visits to their homes. Barring two informants, a Rajput widow and a drunk from the Bhangi caste, everyone in the village was cooperative and responsive. Many helped me cross check the information I needed. As people knew each other well, verification of responses was not a formidable task.

I had 15 key informants. As Vansina (1965) has described, a good informant is one who still lives the customary life, who recalls traditional events and customs readily and enthusiastically, and who is old enough to have acquired some degree of personal experience of his cultural environment. Three men and four women out of the 15 key informants were old, most of them grandparents, with a good knowledge of village traditions, and past and present events and experiences. All the seven were articulate and willing to offer elaborate responses to my queries. The remaining four men and four women informants were younger, aged 18 to 35 years. Although they were less knowledgeable of events pertaining to the remote past they were conversant with the recent past and contemporary conditions. They were well-informed about village youth and their thinking. I developed close relations with the key informants and through them with their households and friends.

In a few weeks of my stay in the village, my presence came to be accepted as a normal phenomenon. People quarrelled and beat children in my presence. Once a man even beat his wife, while I was in their home. During such quarrels, the sequence of recent events surfaced through allegations and counter allegations, and the complexities of family and kin ties got revealed.

Gradually several elderly men and women of all ages came to confide in me. Indifference or denial of help when needed, and non-repayment of debts were the usual complaints in family and neighbourhood disharmonies. Women related as *dērāṇi* and *jēthāṇi* (brothers' wives) and *haoo* and *voo* (mother-in-law and daughter-in-law) called on me separately to pour out their plight. Although I cross checked some of their statements, I never divulged one person's confessions to the other. Probably each one thought that he/she was the only one whose secrets were reposited in me.

Personal relationships with people became a major source of qualitative data. I could be an observer and a participant in events that occurred during the period of fieldwork, while for the events of the past I had to depend on the informants' responses. These responses were described, rationalized and mostly embellished in the idiom of local proverbs, myths, tales and narratives. Songs, stories, dances, games, ceremonies, chants, and cosmological ideas constituted important pieces of data.

In a few months' time it became increasingly clear that old people were important for giving information and for reconstructing past situations regarding which little documented evidence existed. Beals (1955), Chakravarty (1979) and Unni (1979) depended on reports of old respondents to recall historical data in village studies in India. A prolonged debate about the validity and reliability of oral tradition as a source of knowledge owing to a great deal of European prejudice against it is reviewed by Vansina (1965). Steinhart (1989) reiterates Vansina's (1965) observation that oral traditions are a great source of knowledge about the past, particularly among pre-literate people. Nevertheless, Vansina suggests certain practical rules for selecting oral historical material like narratives. For instance, oral traditions should be transmitted by living people and should be supported by similar observations, by social and political conditions, and by chronological corroborations. They should be internally consistent and uncontradicted by people. I followed the above suggestions for the present study.

I observed the behaviour of both old and young people, and noticed that older people were critical of the younger ones' behaviour. Take, for example, the increasing popularity of tea among younger people. Although most of the elderly took more tea than the younger ones, they recalled that they rarely had tea two decades ago. This was corroborated by the few elderly respondents who never took tea. Numerous people confirmed that there was an increase in the number of tea shops and of the customers at them. Adolescent children, especially girls, were even now not allowed to take tea. Similarly young daughters-in-law were rarely offered tea. Parents were considered negligent in their duty if their daughters insisted on having tea which was meant only for grown-ups. A young person, especially a daughter-in-law insisting on tea comes, under sharper criticism as it is a mark of slight disrespect and a sign of independence from senior members of the conjugal household. During the course of my fieldwork, I met a genealogist in his forties, who often recited one of his poems popular for its anti-tea content. The poem portrayed the practice of tea drinking as a milder addiction than opium, and one that spoils health.

I took care to discuss villagers' comments, observations and narrations with some of my key informants. Whenever I found any contradiction I discarded the narration. If several people's narration was similar in description, I sorted out the strand that was common to them.

I had the advantage of observing life in the village for over two decades. I had visited Mogra intermittently since my childhood, though with a long gap in my teens. I could thus recall and cross check several experiences. As a child, I had seen that people did not sell milk, and that butter milk was given generously to the lower castes. But the availability of milk in homes was becoming increasingly scarce with the passage of time. The use of milk in homes had reduced considerably during my fieldwork as compared to the earlier visits. There was thus a ground to feel convinced that the data collected by way of oral history was only marginally influenced by the narrator's personal predisposition and imagination. In order to have an additional experience of village life in the region, I visited several villages in the vicinity of Mogra, namely, Kakani, Shikarpura, Luni, Nimla, Gura and Dhingana.

Some data relevant to the study was obtained from secondary sources as well. A school teacher in Mogra was in charge of maintaining the record of births and deaths. I borrowed these records and duplicated them for my reference. On closer examination, I found several discrepancies between the vital statistical records kept by the village official and my data. Inadequacy in official vital statistics is reported also by Djurfeldt and Lindberg (1976: 46) in their study of a village in south India.

Each census schedule was divided into two major parts which were further divided into a few sections. The first part pertained to the ever married women's identification and their household composition. The second part had sections on marital and reproductive history of the ever married women, their family, landownership, occupation, income and expenditure. The relevance of marital and reproductive history for a meaningful measurement of fertility is rightly suggested by Caldwell (1982) who states that fertility must be analysed over the span of a person's biography. For collecting data on fertility behaviour it was important to reconstruct biographical details of the respondent throught retrospective information and history.

Reconstructing the situations of the people gave a picture of their world and the inner logic of their actions, and what they thought and said. Fieldwork also provided opportunities to see how people come to hold and change their actions and beliefs. Whatever be the importance of reconstructing a person's biographical experience, it was not easy to inquire directly into the marital status of widows and to make the respondents recall deaths of their children. On several occasions, I found women unwilling to talk about their dead children. Some women expressed annoyance at my questions pertaining to their reproductive history. Women aggrieved by the death of a few of their babies and/or grown-up children were the most uncooperative in this regard. At times, even others present during the interview disapproved of questions relating to child deaths, and suggested that I take down names of only the surviving children. Very often, I accepted their suggestion. I returned to the question of child deaths whenever I felt the mother was relatively comfortable with my later questions. Of course, respondents and those surrounding them were relaxed when I met them without paper and pen. I could discuss freely about their dead child(ren) during unstructured interviews (to them, 'gossip'). I managed to cross check the data through key informants, informal meetings with people, and inquiries with neighbours and relatives.

One major hurdle existed regarding the question of marital status. In the village usually this kind of question is not raised, because a woman's dress, ornaments and her overall appearance are sufficient indicators. For instance, as mentioned in Chapter 1, there is a striking contrast between an unmarried and a married girl in the blouses they wear. Similarly, there are subtle differences in jewellery, bangles, and colour of dress between a married woman and a widow, and between women of different castes.

Uniformity in dress is found among girls, both wedded and unwedded. Thus it is common to question whether a particular girl is wedded or not. But the question about a girl's wedding status did not help me because my respondents were to be ever married women. For a teenage girl, the *kānchaḷi* is a sufficient indicator of her 'married' status. The only question then frequently asked is, 'Where (which place) is the girl married off to?' In other words, the inquiry intends to identify the girl's conjugal household and conjugal village. I could distinguish between married and unmarried women in this way. But several elderly women wearing dull coloured *kānchaḷis* and very little jewellery could not be easily distinguished from widows during the initial stage of fieldwork. And there was no conventional way of enquiring about their marital status.

Considering these complications, I inquired about the marital status of most women from their neighbours or relatives prior to my meeting them. I had to make indirect inquiries about the elderly women's husbands' health, age, etc. I either got the answers about the husband, or was told that he was dead. Before I adopted this strategy, I seriously erred in asking a few widows their husband's age, which resulted in awkward situations. The widows responded either by sobbing for having to recollect a tragedy, or by expressing outright anger at such a clumsy question. Of course, one or two of them simply clasified that their husband had passed away. Similarly, the question regarding husband's name could not be addressed to women because a wife is not expected to utter her husband's name. Thus, questions concerning marital status, husband's name and child death had to be modified or raised indirectly during interviews to suit local norms.

Questions pertaining to age, income and expenditure also had to be modified. Senior household members and key informants helped me to collect data on these items. While occupations of respondents and their spouses were recorded fairly easily, those who were too old to work and those who had retired from salaried jobs wer not recorded as 'retired'. Instead the main occupation in which they were engaged for most part of their life was recorded. The same pattern was followed while recording the occupation of the respondent's deceased spouse.

Information pertaining to Mogra as an administrative unit was scrutinized at the Block Development Office in Jodhpur city. Information about the ongoing non-formal and adult education and economic aid programmes for the villages in the region was obtained from the Block Development Office. The information centre called 'Soochna Kendra' and Sumer Public Library at Jodhpur were used for material pertaining to Jodhpur district as well as various villages falling under it. Census publications pertaining to Jodhpur district and carrying information about Mogra were also examined.

APPENDIX 2

# *Glossary*

Only those words occurring more than once in the text are listed here. Diseases listed in Table 5.4 are not.

| | |
|---|---|
| *adūro paḍno* | miscarriage, unintentional premature abortion |
| *adūro patankṇo* | purposeful abortion |
| *āka* | a fistful of grains for alms |
| *ākro vār* | hard day (Sunday, Tuesday) |
| *āṇo* | to bring a bride upon marriage |
| *baccha band karṇo* | stop having children (by sterilization) |
| *bāi, bein* | sister |
| *bajra, bajri* | pearl millet |
| *bapu* | father's father, father's elder brother |
| *bhāg* | fate |
| *bhāi* | brother |
| *Bhākri* | literally, a hillock; Shiva temple on a hillock in Mogra |
| *bhūt* | ghost |
| *bījḷi* | electricity |
| *chautaḷo* | inter-village caste organization |
| *chūrmo* | a sweet made of mashed *roti* (bread) and ghee |
| *dai* | local midwife (usuallyan untouchable) |
| *dāli* | a broad-based basket |
| *dhūḍ avarno,* | a type of magical ritual. |
| *dīlavaḍi* | institution of labour exchange, mostly on farms. |

| | |
|---|---|
| *dūd-roti* | *roti* mashed with milk |
| *dūrviṇ* | telescope |
| *gāgro* | long skirt |
| *gaḷi* | street |
| *gaḷo paḍno* | falling of the throat (believed to be an illness) |
| *gangaji mein ghālno* | immerse the ashes of the deceased in the Ganga |
| *gānv, gaum* | village |
| *gānv ghātḍi* | mortuary feast for village residents |
| *ghar jamāi* | son-in-law resident in his conjugal home |
| *gati* | liberation from the cycle of birth and rebirth, salvation |
| *ghatti* | hand mill |
| *ghee* | clarified butter |
| *ghoḍi* | cradle |
| *gīt gavāṇo* | to sing (in a group), organize group singing |
| *gocher* | common grazing land |
| *Grām Sēwak* | a village-level government employee |
| *gūngto* | veil covering woman's face |
| *hād purāṇo* | attend to a pregnant woman's palate |
| *haḷi* | farm servant employed on annual contract |
| *hanko* | hesitation blended with modesty |
| *hātarvaḍo* | collective ritual mourning |
| *hāto* | marriage by exchange |
| *hāvare melno* | to send to the conjugal home |
| *hīm* | village borders and common land |
| *hiro* | a sweet prepared from ghee, wheat flour, sugar/jaggery and water |
| *hoe* | birth interval between one's children |
| *hōg* | anhedonia, partial mourning |
| *hōgro* | bread made from bajri flour |
| *huāvaḍ* | herbal sweets prepared in ghee for parturient woman |
| *hutak* | Sanskrit, Sutaka; temporary state of impurity |

| | |
|---|---|
| *jagir* | land under *jagirdari* tenure |
| *jagirdari* | a kind of feudal land tenure |
| *jalam bhom* | motherland |
| *jāpa* | woman's confinement |
| *jāpaiti* | a mother in a state of *japa*, post-parturient woman |
| *jati* | caste |
| *jēthāṇi* | husband's elder brother's wife |
| *jīv* | spirit, soul |
| *jīvat sati* | living sati, one who has renounced the world but has not self-immolated |
| *jhāḍa* | a repetitive recitation of a particular mantra by moving one's hand, a twig, or a broom over the ailing person to drive off evil spirit |
| *jōg* | fate |
| *jowar* | a kind of millet |
| *kāchi maut* | untimely death |
| *kād di* | turning out a wife |
| *kāka* | father's younger brother |
| *kāki* | father's younger brother's wife |
| *kānchaḷi* | small blouse worn by ever married women |
| *kanwāra* | virgin, unmarried |
| *kānchaḷi dēṇo* | made to wear a blouse for married woman |
| *kanya dān* | gift of a daughter |
| *karam, karma* | accumulation of good and bad deeds in past life |
| *kaunkaḍ* | see *hīm* |
| *khalsa* | land under direct control of a king |
| *khoḷe bharāvaṇo* | fill the lap, usually with sweets, coconut and cash on ritual occasion |
| *kismat* | fate |
| *lādu* | sweet balls |
| *lāj* | shame |
| *lēk* | fate |
| *lūṇ mirch karṇo* | a magical ritual for driving out evil spirits |

| | |
|---|---|
| *māji* | a term of address for one's mother-in-law |
| *makauṇ* | obligatory mourning visit |
| *moksha* | see *gati* |
| *muklāwo* | consummation of marriage, see also *aṇo* |
| *najar* | evil eye |
| *naṇand* | husband's sister |
| *nasbandi* | sterilization |
| *nāta* | remarriage of widowed or divorced woman |
| *naukri* | salaried job |
| *nyāt* | members of one's caste (*chautaḷo*); large-scale mortuary feast for caste members. |
| *oraṇ* | catchment area for a village pond |
| *ori* | a room to store valuables, clothes, etc., also measles |
| *orno* | half saree, 2–2.5 metres long |
| *pancha* | respectable elders |
| *panchayat* | council |
| *paṇi avārno* | see *dhud avarno* |
| *pannāoḍi* | wedded |
| *pannāvaṇo* | wedding |
| *pāp* | sin |
| *parēj* | physical and dietary restrictions |
| *patwari* | village accountant |
| *pēt balno* | mother's loss of children |
| *pētiyo* | victuals |
| *phaḷo* | main entance to a village settlement |
| *phaura karam* | poor karma |
| *phaura lēk,* | poor fate |
| *pheslo* | verdict |
| *pīḍon raa gāba* | clothes worn by a woman during labour |
| *pīti* | a paste of turmeric powder, water, wheat flour and oil |
| *pittar* | a deceased's spirit placed along other deities in the altar at home |

| | |
|---|---|
| *potiyo* | turban |
| *prēt* | ghost |
| *punna* (*punya*) | religious merit |
| *purdo* | literally, curtain; the institution of women's seclusion |
| *rākhḍi* | amulet prepared by oracles, priests and Brahmins to be tied on the wrists, arms or neck of the ailing |
| *rāḷi* | bed spread stuffed with rags |
| *rilkiyo* | small bed spread |
| *rukāḷo* | protection of fields |
| *sarpanch* | head of statutory village panchayat |
| *sati, satiji* | a widow's self-immolation on her deceased husband's pyre |
| *seenv, seem* | see *hīm* |
| *tābar paḍno* | see *aduro padno* |
| *tābar pataknọ* | see *aduro patakno* |
| *tānko* | underground water storage tank |
| *tānti* | see *rakhḍi* |
| *thān* | small shrine, i.e., spirit centre |
| *thando pēt* | cool womb, indicating no child loss |
| *thuthko nhauknọ* | mimetic spitting meant primarily to ward off evil |
| *ukāḷi* | hot herbal soup, infusion |
| *vāḍa* | cattle shed, patch of land used for cattle and/or storage of fodder |
| *vah* | ward (residential area) |
| *vasti* | housing settlement |
| *vīva* | wedding; see *pannavno* |
| *voo* | daughter-in-law |

APPENDIX 3

# List of Cases

| Name | Sex | Caste | Page |
|---|---|---|---|
| Ajay | M | Charan | 201 |
| Alpu I | F | Patel | 180 |
| Alpu II | F | Patel | 188 |
| Amiya | F | Charan | 155–6 |
| Anadi | F | Kumbar | 79, 81 |
| Anil | M | Charan | 201 |
| Ansi | F | Patel | 112–3, 210 |
| Ansu | F | Charan | 201–2 |
| Baa | M | Patel | 101 |
| Bansoji | M | Sargara | 83 |
| Bijoji | M | Patel | 209 |
| Binja | M | Patel | 201 |
| Bhanwari | F | Bhambi | 207 |
| Bhanwari (Gangu's mother) | F | Jat | 155 |
| Bhera | M | Bhambi | 210 |
| Bhoori | F | Patel | 204–5, 211 |
| Buddha | M | Patel | 87 |
| Chandarki | F | Patel | 89 |
| Chidi | F | Sargara | 212 |
| Chimji | M | Kumbar | 177 |
| Chimu | F | Patel | 75 |
| Choonoji | M | Bhambi | 210 |
| Chuni | F | Patel | 151 |
| Cuki | F | Patel | 79, 81 |
| Dalia | M | Patel | 43 |

| | | | |
|---|---|---|---|
| Mehra | M | Patel | 180 |
| Movni | F | Jat | 102 |
| Nursebenji | F | Brahmin | 113 |
| Paani | F | Patel | 188 |
| Parti | F | Darjee | 96–7, 180 |
| Pemji | M | Raika | 101–2 |
| Phatu | M | Charan | 80 |
| Phatu's wife | F | Charan | 80 |
| Phool | F | Nai | 79 |
| Phooli I | F | Patel | 114 |
| Phooli II | F | Patel | 207 |
| Puni | F | Patel | 102–3 |
| Rajuji | M | Patel | 83 |
| Rambha | F | Raika | 111 |
| Rekha | F | Charan | 80 |
| Roopi | F | Raika | 113 |
| Saori | F | Sargara | 191 |
| Sangari | F | Patel | 192 |
| Satiji | F | Charan | 79 |
| Shera | M | Patel | 140, 201 |
| Shivji | M | Patel | 177 |
| Sona | M | Patel | 148 |
| Sonji | M | Jat | 178 |
| Sugan | F | Charan | 170, 188, 207–8 |
| Sukhi | F | Patel | 111 |
| Umaji | M | Patel | 113 |
| Umaji's wife | F | Patel | 113 |
| Vaddi I | F | Patel | 178 (fn.) |
| Vaddi II | F | Patel | 205, 211–2 |
| Vanji | M | Sargara | 210 |
| Vaski | F | Patel | 170 |
| Veeri | F | Darjee | 210 |
| Vena | M | Patel | 205 |
| Vijaji | M | Patel | 177–8 |
| Vinji | F | Patel | 100–101 |

Total number of cases = 98, Female 64, Male 34

# Bibliography


Aden, A. and Birk, S.
1981 A Study of Child Mortality in Mogadishu, Somalia, *Journal of Tropical Pediatrics*, 27(6): 279–84.

Afshar, H (ed.)
1985 *Women, Work and Ideology in the Third World*, London: Tavistock.

Agarwala, S. N.
1966a *Some Problems of India's Population*, Bombay: Vora.

1966b Raising the Marriage Age for Women: A Means to Lower the Birth Rate, *Economic and Political Weekly*, 1: 797–8.

1970 *A Demographic Study of Six Urbanising Villages*, New York: Asia.

Alexander, P.
1984 Women, Labour and Fertility: Population Growth in 19th Century Java, *Mankind*, 14: 361–72.

Anker, R.
1977 The effect of Group Level Variables on Fertility in a Rural Indian Sample, *Journal of Development Studies*. 14(1): 63–77.

Anker, R. and Anker, M.
1982 *Reproductive Behaviour in the Households of Rural Gujarat*, New Delhi: Concept.

Arnold, F. *et al*.
1975 *The Value of Children: A Cross-National Study*. vol. 1, Honolulu: East-West Population Institute.

Atal, Y.
1968 *Changing Frontiers of Caste*, New Delhi: National.

Bailey, F. G.
1957 *Caste and the Economic Frontier*, Manchester: Manchester University Press.

Bailey, F. G.
1959 For a Sociology of India? *Contributions to Indian Sociology*, III: 88–101.
Beals, A. R.
1955 Interplay among Factors of Change in a Mysore Village, in M. Marriott (ed.), *Village India*, Chicago: University of Chicago Press.
Bebarta, P. C.
1966 Family Type and Fertility, *Economic and Political Weekly*, 1: 633–4.
Becker, G. S.
1960 An Economic Analysis of Fertility, in *Demographic and Economic Change in Developed Countries*, Princeton: Princeton University Press.

1965 A Theory of the Allocation of Time, *Economic Journal*, 75 (September): 493–517.
Beliwinkel, M.
1979 Objective Appreciation through Subjective Involvement, in M. N. Srinivas, A. M. Shah and E. A. Ramaswamy (eds.), *The Fieldworker and the Field*, Delhi: Oxford University Press.
Benedict, B.
1970 Population Regulation in Primitive Societies, in A. Allision (ed.), *Population Control*, Baltimore: Penguin.
Berger, P.
1969 *The Social Reality of Religion*, Harmondsworth: Penguin.
Berger, P. and Luckman, T.
1967 *The Social Construction of Reality*, Harmondsworth: Penguin.
Bernstein, B.
1977 *Class, Codes and Control*, vol. 3, London: Routledge and Kegan Paul.
Beteille, A. and Madan, T. N. (eds.),
1975 *Encounter and Experience*, Delhi: Vikas.
Bhatia, B. M.
1963 *Famines in India*, London: Asia.
Birdsall, N. and Jamison, D. T.
1983 Income and Other Factors Influencing Fertility in China, *Population and Development Review*, 9(4): 651–75.

Bloch, I. E. D.
1908 *The Sexual Life of Our Time in its Relations to Modern Civilization*, New York: Rebman.
Bongaarts, J.
1978 A Framework for Analysing the Proximate Determinants of Fertility, *Population and Development Review*, 4 (1): 105–32.
Bose, A.
1988 *From Population to People*, vol. 1, Delhi: B. R. Publishing.
Bose, A., Desai, P. B., Mitra, A. and Sharma, J. N.
1974 *Population in India's Development—1947–2000*, Delhi: Vikas.
Bose, A. B. and Jodha, N. S.
1965 The Jajmani System in a Desert Village, *Man in India*, 45: 105–26.
Bose, A. B. and Jodha, N. S. and Malhotra, S. P.
1964 Studies in Group Dynamics: Factionalism in a Desert Village, *Man in India*, 44: 311–28.
Bulatao, R. A. and Lee, R. D. (eds.)
1983 *Determinants of Fertility in Developing Countries*. New York: Academic Press.
Cain, M.
1977 The Economic Activities of Children in a Village in Bangladesh, *Population and Development Review*, 3: 201–27.

1981 Risk and Fertility in India and Bangladesh, *Population and Development Review*, 7: 435–74.
Cain, M., Khanam, S. R. and Nahar, S.
1979 Class, Patriarchy and Women's Work in Bangladesh, *Population and Development Review*, 5(3): 405.
Caldwell, J. C.
1976 Fertility and the Household Economy in Nigeria, *Journal of Comparative Family Studies*, 7: 193–253.

1982 *Theory of Fertility Decline*, London: Academic Press.
Caldwell, J. C. and Caldwell, P.
1977 The Role of Marital Sexual Abstinence in Determining Fertility: A Study of the Yoruba in Nigeria, *Population Studies*, 31: 193–217.

Caldwell, J. C. and Cladwell, P.
1981 The Function of Child-spacing in Traditional Societies and the Direction of Change, in H.J. Page, and R. Lesthaeghe (eds.), *Child Spacing in Tropical Africa: Traditions and Change*, London: Academic Press.

Caldwell, J. C., Reddy, P. H. and Caldwell, P.
1984 Determinants of Fertility Decline in Rural South India, in T. Dyson and N. Crook (eds.), *India's Demography*, New Delhi: South Asian.

Caldwell, J. C., Caldwell, P. and Caldwell, B.
1987 Anthropology and Demography: The Mutual Reinforcement of Speculation and Research, *Current Anthropology*, 28(1): 25–43.

Carr-Saunders, A. M.
1922 *The Population Problem: A Study in Human Evolution*, Oxford: Clarendon Press.

Cassen, R.
1975 Welfare and Population: Notes on Rural India Since 1960, *Population and Development Review*, 1(1): 33–70.

1978 *India: Population, Economy, Society*, London: Macmillan.

Census of India
1971 *General Population Tables*, Series 1, Part II A(i), New Delhi: Registrar-General and Census Commissioner of India.

1981a *Primary Census Abstract: General Population*, Series 1, India, Part II, B(i), New Delhi: Registrar-General and Census Commissioner of India.

1981b *Report and Tables Based on 5 Percent Sample Data*, Series 1, India, Part II Special, New Delhi: Registrar-General and Census Commissioner of India.

1981c *District Census Handbook—Jodhpur*, Jaipur: Director of Census Operations, Rajasthan.

1981d *Household Population by Religion of Head of Household*, Series 1, Paper 4 of 1984, New Delhi: Registrar-General and Census Commissioner of India.

Chakravarti, A.
1975 *Contradiction and Change*, Delhi: Oxford University Press.

1979 Experiences of an Encapsulated Observer, in Srinivas, Shah and Ramaswamy, (1979: 38–57).

Chandrasekaran, C.
1986 Cultural Emphasis in the Mysore Population Study, in K. Mahadevan (ed.), *Fertility and Mortality*, New Delhi: Sage.

Chandrasekaran, C. and George, M. V.
1962 Mechanisms Underlying the Differences in Fertility Patterns of Bengalee Women from three Socio-economic Groups, *Milbank Memorial Fund Quarterly*, 40: 59–89.

Charles, N. and Kerr, M.
1988 *Women, Food and Families*, Manchester: Manchester University Press.

Chauhan, B. R.
1967 *A Rajasthan Village*, New Delhi: Vir.

Coale, A. J. and Hoover, E. M.
1958 *Population Growth and Economic Development in Low Income Countries*, Princeton: Princeton University Press.

Conklin, G. H.
1976 Family Structure, Caste and Economic Development—Rural Comparison From Dharwar, in G. R. Gupta (ed.), *Family and Social Change in Modern India*. Delhi: Vikas.

Dandekar, K.
1959 *Demographic Survey of Six Rural Communities*, Bombay: Asia.

Das, V.
1977 *Structure and Cognition*, Delhi: Oxford University Press.

Das Gupta, M.
1987 Selective Discrimination Against Female Children in Rural Punjab, India, *Population and Development Review*, 13(i): 77–100.

Datta, K. K. *et al.*
1980 Morbidity Pattern Among Rural Pregnant Women in Alwar, Rajasthan—A Cohort Study, *Health and Population: Perspectives and Issues*, 3(4): 282–93.

Davis, K. and Blake, J.
1956 Social Structure and Fertility: An Analytical Framework, *Economic Development and Cultural Change*, 4(3): 211–35.

Demeny, P.
1981 Research on the Determinants of Fertility: A Note on Priorities, *Population and Development Review*, 7(2): 311–24.
Djurfeldt, G. and Lindberg, S.
1976 *Pills Against Poverty*, New Delhi: Oxford and IBH.
Douglas, M.
1960 *Purity and Danger*. Edition used, 1979. London: Routledge and Kegan Paul.

1966 Population Control in Primitive Groups, *British Journal of Sociology*, 17: 263–73.
Driver, E. D.
1963 *Differential Fertility in Central India*, Princeton: Princeton University Press.
Dube, L.
1986 Seed and Earth: The Symbolism of Biological Reproduction and Sexual Relations in Reproduction, in L. Dube, E. Lealock and S. Arderner (eds.), *Visibility and Power*, Delhi: Oxford University Press.
Dube, S. C.
1955 *Indian Village*, Newyork: Cornell University Press.
Dumont, L.
1970 *Homo Hierarchicus*, London: Weidenfeld and Nicolson.
Dumont, L. and Pocock, D. F.
1957 Village Studies, *Contributions to Indian Sociology*, 1: 23–42.
Durkheim, E.
1912 *The Elementary Forms of Religious Life*, Edition used, 1964, London: Allen and Unwin.
Easterlin, R. A.
1975 An Economic Framework of Fertility Analysis, *Studies in Family Planning*, 6: 54–63.
Endres, M. E.
1975 *On Defusing the Population Bomb*, Cambridge, Mass: Halstead Press.
Engels, F.
1884 *The Origin of the Family, Private Property and the State*, Edition used, 1972, London: Lawrence and Wishart.
Enke, S.
1966 The Economic Aspects of Slowing Population Growth, *Economic Journal*, 76: 44–56.

Epstein, T. S. and Jackson, D. (eds.)
1975 *Paradox of Poverty*, Delhi: Macmillan.

Erikson, E. H.
1950 *Childhood and Society*, Edition used, 1972, Harmondsworth: Penguin.

Fawcett, J. T.
1970 *Psychology and Population*, New York: Population Council.

1976 The Value and Cost of First Child, Paper presented at the Conference on the First Child, Asilomar, California.

1986 The Value and Cost of Children: Converging Theory and Research, *In* Mahadevan (1986: 65–84).

Fawcett, J. T. (ed.)
1972 *The Satisfactions and Costs of Children: Theories, Concepts, Methods*, Honolulu: East-West Population Institute.

Firth, R.
1963 *We, the Tikopia: A Sociological Study of Kinship in Primitive Polynesia*, Boston: Beacon Press.

Fortes, M.
1958 Introduction, *In* J. Goody (ed.), *The Developmental Cycle of the Domestic Groups*, Cambridge: Cambridge University Press.

Frake, C. O.
1973 The Diagnosis of Disease among the Subanun of Mindanao, in N. Keddie (ed.), *Tinker Tailor: The Myth of Cultural Deprivation*, Harmondsworth: Penguin.

Freebeme, M.
1964 Birth Control in China, *Population Studies*, 18(1): 5–16.

Freedman, R.
1963 *The Sociology of Human Fertility: A trend Report and Bibliography*, Oxford: Basil Blackwell.

1975 *The Sociology of Human Fertility: Annotated Bibliography*, New York: Irvington Press.

1979 Theories of Fertility Decline: A Reappraisal, *Social Forces*, 58: 1–17.

Gaiha, R.
1982 *On Measuring the Risk of Poverty in Rural India*, Delhi: Faculty of Management Studies, University of Delhi, Mimeo.

George, S.
1976 *How the Other Half Dies*, Harmondsworth: Penguin.

Giddens, A.
1984 *The Constitution of Society*, Cambridge: Polity Press.

Gould, H.
1969 Sex and Contraception in Sherpur: Family in a North Indian Village, *Economic and Political Weekly*, 4: 1887–92.

Greer, G.
1984 *Sex and Destiny*, London: Secker and Warburg.

Gupta, K. A.
1979 Travails of a Woman Fieldworker, in Srinivas, Shah and Ramaswamy (1979: 103–14).

Handwerker, W. P.
1983 The First Demographic Transition: An Analysis of Substantive Choices and Reproductive Consequences, *American Anthropologist*, 85: 5–27.

Handwerker, W. P. (ed.)
1986 *Culture and Reproduction*, Boulder and London: Westview Press.

1986 "Natural Fertility" as a Balance of Choice and Behavioural Effect: Policy Implications for Liberian Farm Households, *In* Handwerker (1986: 90–111).

Hawthorn, G.
1970 *The Sociology of Fertility*, London: Collier-MacMillan.

Heer, D. M.
1964 Fertility Differentials between Indian and Spanish Speaking Parts of Andean Countries, *Population Studies*, 18(1): 71–84.

1972 *Determinants of Family Planning Attitudes and Practices*, Cambridge, Mass.: Harvard University.

Howell, N.
1979 *Demography of the Dobe! Kung*. New York: Academic Press.

Illich, I.
1975 *Medical Nemesis*, Calcutta: Rupa.

Jain, S. P.
1975 *Demography: A Status Study of Population Research in India*, vol. II, New Delhi: Tata McGraw Hill.

Jain, S. P. and Visaria, P. (eds.)
1988 *Infant Mortality in India*, New Delhi: Sage.

Jeffery, R., *et al.*
1984 Only Cord Cutters? Midwifery and Childbirth in Rural North India, *Social Action*, 34(3): 229–50.

Jodha, N. S.
1985 Market Forces and Erosion of Common Property Resources, in Agricultural Markets in the Semi-arid Tropics, Proceedings of the international workshop, ICRISAT Centre, Patancheru, Andhra Pradesh, India. 24–8 October.

Jordan, B.
1980 *Birth in Four Cultures: A Cross-Cultural Investigation of Childbirth in Yucatan, Holland, Sweden and the United States*, Montreal: Eden Press.

Joshi, P. C.
1979 Fieldwork Experience: Relived and Reconsidered, in Srinivas, Shah and Ramaswamy (1979: 73–99).

Kabeer, N.
1985 Do Women Gain from High Fertility? in H. Afshar (ed.), *Women, Work and Ideology in the Third World*, London: Tavistock.

Kanitkar, T. and Murthy, B. N.
1988 Factors Associated with Infant Mortality in Rajasthan and Orissa, in A. K. Jain and P. Visaria (1988: 297–321).

Kara, P. K. and Sinha, B. N.
1987 Family Welfare Programme and its Evaluation: Implications and Recommendations, in R. N. Pati (ed.), *Population, Family and Culture*. New Delhi: Ashish.

Karve, I.,
1965 *Kinship Organisation in India*, second ed., Bombay: Asia.

Khan, M. E. *et al.*
1983 Women and Health—A Case Study of Sex Discrimination, Paper presented at the Joint ICMR-Ford Foundation Workshop on Child Health, Nutrition and Family Planning, Bangalore.

Kirk, D.
1971 A New Demographic Transition, in *Rapid Population Growth: Consequences and Policy Implications*, Baltimore: John Hopkins Press.

Kitzingr, S.
1982 Social Context of Birth: Some Comparisons between Childbirth in Jamaica and Britain, in C. P. MacCormack (ed.), *Ethnography of Fertility and Birth*, London: Academic Press.

Kohli, K. L.
1977 *Mortality in India*, Delhi: Sterling.

Kolenda, P.
1968 Region, Caste and Family Structure: A Comparative Study of the Indian Joint Family, in M. Singer and B. S. Cohn (eds.), *Structure and Change in Indian Society*, New York: Wenner-Gren Foundation for Anthropological Research.

1989 The Joint Family Household in Rural Rajasthan: Ecological, Cultural and Demographic Conditions for its Occurrence, in J. .N. Gray and D. J. Mearns (eds.), *Society From the Inside Out*, New Delhi: Sage.

Krause, E.
1980 *Why Study Sociology*?, New York: Random House.

Kunstadter, P.
1984 Cultural Ideals, Socioeconomic Change and Household Composition, in M. R. Netting, R. R. Wilk, and E. J. Arnould (eds.), *Households: Comparative and Historical Studies of the Domestic Group*, Berkeley: University of California Press.

Laderman, C.
1983 *Wives and Midwives*, Berkeley: University of California Press.

Lancaster, K. J.
1966 A New Approach to Consumer Theory, *Journal of Political Economy*, 74 (April): 132–57.

Leach, E.
1976 *Culture and Communication: The Logic by which Symbols are Connected*. Cambridge University Press.

Lealock, E.
1986 Women, Power and Authority, *Journal of Poltical Economy*, 74 (April): 132–57.

Leibenstein, H.
1981 Economic Decision Theory and Human Fertility Behaviour: A Speculative Essay, *Population and Development Review*, 7(3): 381–400.

Leiberman, S. S.
1980 Rural Development and Fertility Transition in South Asia: A Case for Broad Based Strategy, *Social Research*, 47(2): 305–38.
Levi-Strauss, C.
1966 *The Savage Mind*, Chicago: University of Chicago Press.
Lipton, M.
1984 Household Size and Poverty, in Dyson and Crook (1984: 209–34).
Lewis, O.
1958 *Village Life in North India*, Urbana: University of Illinois Press.
Lorimer, F.
1954 *Culture and Human Fertility: A Study of the Relation of Culture Conditions to Fertility in Non-Industrial and Transitional Societies*, Paris: Unesco.
MacCormack, C. P. (ed.)
1982 *Ethnography of Fertility and Birth*, London: Academic Press.
Madan, T. N.
1987 *Non-Renunciation*, New Delhi: Oxford University Press.
Mahadevan, K. *et al.*
1981 Culture, Nutrition and Infant and Child Mortality: A Study in South Central India, Paper presented at the general conference of IUSSP, Manila.
Mahadevan, K. and Sumangala, M.
1987 *Social Development, Cultural Change and Fertility Decline*, New Delhi: Sage.
Mahobia, K.
1976 *Bikaner Rajya Mein Ganvon Ka Swaroop (Satrahveen, Atharveen Shatabdi mein)*, Hindi, Jaipur: Rajasthan History Congress, Proceedings vol. VIII, Ajmer session 1975: 11–9.
Malinowski, B.
1948 *Magic, Science and Religion and Other Essays*, London: Souvenir Press.
Mamadani, M.
1972 *The Myth of Population Control*, New York: Monthly Review Press.
Mandelbaum, D. G.
1970 *Society in India*, Bombay: Popular.

Mandelbaum, D. G.
1974 *Human Fertility in India*, Berkeley: University of California Press.

Mathen, K. K.
1962 Preliminary Lessons Learned from the Rural Population Control Study of Singur, in C. V. Kiser (ed.), *Research in Family Planning*, Princeton: Princeton University Press.

Mauldin, W. P. and Berelson, B.
1978 Conditions of Fertility Decline in Developing Countries, 1965–75. *Studies in Family Planning*, 9(5): 90–147.

McKintosh, M.
1981 The Sexual Division of Labour and the Subordination of Women, in K. Yong, C. Wolkowitz and R. McCullagh (eds.), *Of Marriage and the Market*. London: CSE Books.

Meillassoux, C.
1991 *The Anthropology of Slavery*, London: The Athlone Press.

Minocha, A.
1979 Varied Roles in the Field, in Srinivas, Shah and Ramaswamy (1979: 201–15).

Miro, C. A. and Potter, J. E.
1980 *Population Policy: Research Priorities in the Developing World*, London: Frances Pinter.

Mosley, W. H. (ed.)
1977 *Nutrition and Human Reproduction*, Washington, D. C.: National Institute of Health.

Mueller, E.
1972 Economic Motives for Family Limitation: A Study Conducted in Taiwan, *Population Studies*, 26(3): 323–403.

Nag, M.
1972 Sex, Culture and Human Fertility: India and the United States, *Current Anthropology*, 13: 231–7, 260–3.

Nag, M., Peet, R. C. and White, B. N. F.
1978 An Anthropological Approach to the Study of the Economic Value of Children in Java and Nepal, *Current Anthropology*, 19: 293–306.

Namboodiri, N. K.
1986 Social Development and Population Change: A Reappraisal of Selected Theories, in Mahadevan (1986: 37–54).

Notestein, F. W.
1945 Population: The Long View, in T. W. Shultz (ed.), *Food for the World*, Chicago: University of Chicago Press.

Opler, M. E.
1964 Cultural Context and Population Control Programmes in Village India, in E. W. Count and G. Bowles (eds.), *Fact and Theory in Social Science*, Syracuse: Syracuse University Press.

Page, H. J. and Lesthaeghe, R. (eds.)
1967 *Child Spacing in Tropical Africa: Traditions and Change*, London: Academic Press.

Pakrasi, K. and Malaker, C.
1967 The Relationship between Family Type and Fertility, *Milbank Memorial Fund Quarterly*, 45: 451–60.

Papanek, H.
1973 Men, Women and Work: Reflections on the Two Person Career, in J. Huber (ed.), *Changing Women in a Changing Society*, Chicago: University of Chicago Press.

Parish, W. L. and Whyte, M. K.
1978 *Village and Family in Contemporary China*, Chicago: University of Chicago Press.

Patel, T.
1982 Domestic Group, Status of Women, and Fertility, *Social Action*, 32(4): 363–79.

1987 Women's Work and their Status: Dialectics of Subordination and Assertion, *Social Action*, 37(2): 126–49.

Pebley, A. R. *et al.*
1979 Fertility Desires and Child Mortality Experience among Guatemalan Women, *Studies in Family Planning*, 10(4): 135.

Pocock, D. F.
1962 Notes on Jajmani Relationship, *Contributions to Indian Sociology*, 6: 78–95.

Poffenberger, T.
1969 *Husband-Wife Communication and Motivational Aspects of Population Control in an Indian Village*, New Delhi: Central Family Planning Institute Monograph Series, No. 10.

Pohlman, E.
1969 *The Psychology of Birth Planning*, Cambridge, Mass: Schenkman.

Polgar, S. (ed.)
1971 *Culture and Population: A Collection of Current Studies*, Cambridge: Schenkman.

Poti, S. J. and Dutta, S.
1960 Pilot Study on Social Mobiity and Differential Fertility, *Studies in Family Planning*, New Delhi: Director-General of Health Services.

Potter, R. G.
1963 Birth Intervals: Structure and Change, *Population Studies*, 17(2): 155–66.

Potter, R. G. and Parker, M. P.
1964 Predicting the Time Required to Conceive, *Population Studies*, 18(1): 99–116.

Prabhakara, N. R. and Usha, M. N.
1986 *Population Growth and Unemployment in India*, New Delhi: Ashish.

Rajasthan Rajya Pathyapustak Mandal (RRPM)
1984a *Samajik Gyan, Kaksha,* 7, Hindi, Edition used, 1984–7, Jaipur: R. K. Printers.

1984b *Samajik Gyan, Kaksha 8*, Hindi, Edition used, 1984–7. Chandigarh: Akal Printers.

1984c *Samajik Gyan- 1 [Bhugole], Kaksha 8*, Hindi, Edition used, 1984–8, Jullundhar: Jullundhar Cooperative.

Ramu, G. N.
1988 *Family Structure and Fertility*, New Delhi: Sage.

Rao, K. G.
1974 *Studies in Family Planning: India*, New Delhi: Abhinav.

Rao, M. N. and Mathen, K. K.
1970 *Rural Field Study of Population Control, Singur*, Calcutta: All India Institute of Hygiene and Public Health.

Registrar-General, India
1983 *Survey on Infant and Child Mortality, 1979*, Delhi: Office of the Registrar-General, India.

Rele, J. R.
1963 Fertility Differentials in India—Evidence from a Rural Background, *Milbank Memorial Fund Quarterly*, 41: 183–97.

Repetto, R.
1979 *Economic Equality and Fertility in Developing Countries*, Baltimore: John Hopkins University Press.

Ruzicka, L. T.
1984 Mortality in India: Past Trends and Future Prospects, in Dyson and Crook (1984: 13–36).

Ryder, J. W.
1976 Interrelations Between Family Structure and Fertility in Yucatan, in B. A. Kaplan (ed.), *Anthropological Studies of Human Fertility*, Michigan: Wayne State University Press.

Sahlins, M.
1972 *Stone-Age Economics*, Chicago: Aldine-Atherton.

Schapera, I.
1955 An Anthropologist's Approach to Population Growth: Studies in the Bechuanaland Protectorate, in J. B. Cragg and N. W. Pirie (eds), *The Numbers of Men and Animals*, Edinburgh: Oliver and Boyd.

Shah, A. M.
1973 *The Household Dimension of the Family in India*, Delhi: Orient Longman.

Shah, A. M. and Desai, I. P.
1988 *Division and Hierarchy: An Overview of Caste in Gujarat*, Delhi: Hindustan.

Shah, A. M., Desai, I. P. and Shroff, R. G.
1958 The Vahivancha Barots of Gujarat: A Case of Genealogists and Mythographers, *Journal of American Folkore*, (281): 246–8.

Sharma, K. L.
1974 *The Changing Rural Stratification System*, New Delhi: Orient Longman.

Singh, K. P.
1986 *Correlates of Fertility Behaviour*, New Delhi: Concept.

Smith, T. C.
1977 *Nakahara: Family Planning and Population in a Japanese Village, 1717–1830*, Stanford: Stanford University Press.

Sontag, S.
1979 *Illness as Metaphor*, New York: Vintage.

Srinivas, M. N.
1952 *Religion and Society among the Coorgs of South India*, Oxford: Clarendon Press.

1955 The Social System of a Mysore Village, in M. Marriott, (ed.), *Village India*, Chicago: University of Chicago Press.

1959 The Dominant Caste in Rampura, *American Anthropologist*, 61: 1–16.

1965 *India: Social Structure*, Edition used, 1982, Delhi: Hindustan.

Srinivas, M. N.
1975 The Indian Village: Myth and Reality, in J. M. Beattie (ed.), *Evans-Pritchard Festschrift*, Oxford: Clarendon Press.

1978 Village Studies, Participant Observation and Social Science Research in India, in B. Das Gupta (ed.), *Village Studies in the Third World*, Delhi: Hindustan.

Srinivas, M. N. and Ramaswamy, E. A.
1977 *Culture and Human Fertility in India*, New Delhi: Oxford University Press.

Srinivas, M. N., Shah, A. M. and Ramaswamy, E. A. (eds.)
1979 *The Fieldworker and the Field*, Delhi: Oxford University Press.

Srinivasan, K.
1986 Modernisation and Fertility Change: A Review of Theoretical Developments, in Mahadevan (1986: 171–83).

Srinivasan, K. and Kanitkar, T.
1984 The Contrasting Demography of Bihar and Rajasthan: Findings from Recent Sample Surveys, in Dyson and Crook (1984: 73–91).

Stroebe, W. and Stroebe, M. S.
1987 *Bereavement and Health*, Cambridge: Cambridge University Press.

Steinhart, E. I.
1989 Introduction, *Ethnohistory*, 36(1): 1–8.

Stephens, M.
1986 Childbirth Industry: A Woman's View, in Dube, Lealock and Arderner (1986: 70–83).

Talwar, P. P.
1988 Infant Mortality: Some Evidence from Rural Madhya Pradesh, in Jain and Visaria (1988: 323–38).

Thompson, W.
1929 Population, *American Journal of Sociology*, 34: 959–75.

Tilly, C.
1978 The Historical Study of Vital Processes, in C. Tilly (ed.), *Historical Studies of Changing Fertility*, Princeton: University Press.

Tod, J.
1920 *Annals and Antiquities of Rajasthan*, London: Oxford University Press.

United Nations
1961 *The Mysore Population Study: A Cooperative Project of United Nations and the Government of India*, New York.

1973 *Determinants and Consequences of Population Trends*, New York.

1974 *Concise Report on the World Population Situation in 1970–75*, New York.

1981 *Variations in the Incidence of Knowledge and Use of Contraception: A Comparative Analysis of World Fertility Survey Results of Twenty Developing Countries*, New York.

Unni, K. R.
1979 On Tracks and Tracts in My Fieldwork, in Srinivas, Shah and Ramaswamy (1979: 58–72).

Van Gennep, A.
1960 *The Rites of Passage*, Chicago: University of Chicago Press.

Vansina, J.
1965 *Oral Tradition: A Study in Historical Methodology*, London: Routledge and Kegan Paul.

Visaria, P.
1980 *Poverty and Living Standards in Asia*, Working Paper No. 2, Washington: World Bank.

Visaria, L.
1988 Levels, Trends and Determinants of Infant Mortality in India, in Jain and Visaria (1988: 67–126).

White, B.
1975 The Economic Importance of Children in a Javanese Village, in M. Nag (ed.), *Population and Social Organisation*, The Hague, Paris: Mouton.

1976 Population Involution and Employment in Rural Java, *Development and Change*, 7: 267–90.

Wilson, C.
1984 Natural Fertility in Pre-industrial England, 1600–1799. *Population Studies*, 38: 225–40.

Wiser, W. H.
1936 *The Hindu Jajmani System*, Lucknow: Lucknow.

Wiser, W. H. and Wiser, C.
1963 *Behind Mud Walls*, 1930–1960, Berkeley: University of California Press.

Wolf, E. R.
1969 *Peasant Wars of the Twentieth Century*, New York: Harper and Row.

Wyon, J. B. and Gordon, J. E.
1971 *The Khanna Study*, Cambridge, Mass.: Harvard University Press.

# Index